God Still Heals

God Still Heals

*Answers to Your Questions
about Divine Healing*

James L. Garlow
and
Carol Jane Garlow

wesleyan
publishing
house

Indianapolis, Indiana

© 2005 by James L. Garlow and Carol Jane Garlow. All rights reserved.
Published by Wesleyan Publishing House
Indianapolis, Indiana 46250
Printed in the United States of America

ISBN-13: 978-0-89827-295-6   *God Still Heals*
ISBN-10: 0-89827-295-5   *God Still Heals*
ISBN-13: 978-0-89827-316-8   *God Still Heals* with CD *The Healing*
ISBN-10: 0-89827-316-1   *God Still Heals* with CD *The Healing*

Dedicated to

John Wimber
1934–1997

Who, among many other things, was
a healer and a teacher of healing, and
whose thumbprint is on much of this book

———∞∞———

Also lovingly dedicated to four groups of persons—

To the many who have struggled with disease
and have received healing—we rejoice with
you

To the many who have struggled with disease
and have not yet received healing—we continue
to pray for you

To the many who were prayed for repeatedly
yet did not receive healing before graduating
to heaven—we will not forget you

To the many grieving loved ones left behind—
we weep with you

"I have heard your prayer; I have seen your tears. Behold, I will heal you."

—II Kings 20:5

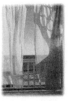

CONTENTS

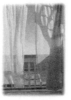

PREFACE

This book is your invitation to pray for, expect, and experience the gift of divine healing. Understandably, many people are skeptical of the notion that God continues to miraculously heal people in our day. Frustrated by a lack of result in spite of faithful prayer, many have concluded that God is either unable or unwilling to heal those who call upon him. It is true that many aspects of divine healing remain a mystery, and for reasons we may never comprehend, some people are not made well.

Yet God still heals.

We have seen evidence of his healing power around us, and we have experienced that healing ourselves. We are aware that many who will read this book have suffered with illness and pain for many years. Having experienced significant illness ourselves, we have great sympathy for those who are suffering. It is our desire that the words of this book may bring encouragement—never condemnation—to those who suffer. The purpose of this book is simply to call the church to pray expectantly for healing so that the sick shall be made well. To all, we humbly extend an invitation to seek God's healing power.

We believe strongly in the power of prayer. There is no more effective means of praying than to pray the words of Scripture. Appendix A contains a number of Scripture-based prayers. Use these prayers as a guide as you begin to pray Scripture. In time you may begin to compose your own Scripture prayers, or simply use the Scripture text as your prayer book.

Each of the chapters in this book begins with a story. All of the stories are fictionalized, although some of them are based on life experiences. Two of the stories involve us personally, and those are noted in the text. In all other cases, the people and events are fictitious.

———— ❧ ————

Over the years a number of people have influenced my thinking on the subject of divine healing. First among them is John Wimber.

In early 1983 my friend John Patredis handed me a copy of *Christian Life* magazine with an unusual cover article titled simply "MC510." That symbol was the course designation for a class at Fuller Theological Seminary called "Signs, Wonders, and Church Growth." The course was largely taught by John Wimber under the supervision of Dr. C. Peter Wagner.

The cover story told of Wimber, a Southern California pastor, who taught about healing and praying for the sick in, of all things, a seminary class. Over the years, I had heard many people say that they had been healed with no evidence to support the claim. I had also seen television preachers claim that people were healed without any substantive proof. Although I was open to the concept of healing as a truly biblical notion, I did not have enough understanding to actually engage in praying for the sick. I had longed to see God's healing power released in our day as it had been in the past. That is exactly what was described in the article "MC510." According to this report, people were actually being healed, complete with medical confirmation.

Hungry to experience God's presence and power, I decided to travel from Dallas–Ft. Worth, where I was living at the time, to Anaheim, California, to attend a one-week version of the class. That would be the beginning of a significant change in my life. I became, as I call it, "Wimber-ized."

Over two decades have passed since then. The passage of time has allowed my thinking to season, and that is a great advantage. A disadvantage, however, is that over the years important notes and tapes of John Wimber's teaching have been lost or misplaced. As a result, I am unable to appropriately document a number of ideas that I am sure originated with Wimber. It is now difficult for me to tell where the teacher (John Wimber) leaves off and the student (Jim Garlow) begins. He shaped my understanding of divine healing, and I regret that I cannot precisely identify his original ideas.

For that reason, I have dedicated this book to John Wimber. His thoughts were so stamped on my mind that they are, in more ways than I may be aware, found on the following pages. If any of the teachings in this book sound like something John Wimber might have said, that could be because he did. Without his influence on my life, this book would never have come into being. Much of my understanding of healing came from this great man of God. I gratefully acknowledge John Wimber's influence on my life, and I humbly dedicate this book to him.

Although I wrote most of this book, my co-author, wife, confidant, and ministry colleague, Carol Garlow, knows more about healing than I ever will. Whereas I have healing "fruit" from my brief prayers for people at the weekend services at Skyline Wesleyan Church, Carol prays for the sick for hours at a time in powerful weekly healing services. Her primary contributions to this book are the chapter on the relationship between worship and healing, and the Scripture-based prayers comprised in the appendix. I have learned much from her insistence on praying the Word, and I have learned much more from her steadfast, unwavering confidence in God.

The intercessors on Carol's team are exceptionally gifted, insightful, and persistent prayer warriors. Their quiet and unsung faithfulness has blessed many on Wednesday nights at the healing class, on weekends in the healing tent, and in other times and places that we may never know about. Their past willingness to make "healing house calls" on a consistent basis and to comprise the spiritual care network of a local hospital makes them unique.

Influencing me greatly in my healing journey are two powerful prayer warriors: Judy Garlow Wade, my sister, and her husband, Keat Wade. They have become prayer leaders across our city, around our state, and across our nation. Judy's book *Take the Name of Jesus With You,* is a picture of what it means to contagiously carry Jesus' power into the most difficult situations. Keat and Judy's faith in God convicts me; their understanding of Him inspires me.

Along the way, a number of other people have touched my life on this topic.

The late Merlin Budy, an Alva, Oklahoma, wheat farmer, persuaded me to have a greater expectation of the miraculous.

A 1983 talk by Charles Capps, a cotton farmer from England, Arkansas, sent me scurrying to the Scriptures to study faith and healing.

A three day seminar, *In the Word,* by the late Milton Green, a carpet cleaner from Cleveland, Tennessee, made me aware of the power of the Word of God.

A book by Don Basham entitled *Deliver Us from Evil* initially opened my eyes to the issue of deliverance.

A book by Francis McNutt called *Healing* helped me overcome my fear of praying for the sick.

Evangelist James Robinson's journey with Jesus spilled over on me and caused me to become more passionate about Christ.

Each of these, along with many others, shaped much of my thinking on healing and my practice of praying for the sick. Be assured that their insights are sprinkled throughout these pages.

As I made my journey into healing, two congregations helped and encouraged me a great deal.

The people of Metroplex Chapel (Church of the Nazarene), a church in the heart of Dallas–Ft. Worth that I had the joy of planting in 1983 and pastoring for thirteen years, were courageous enough to become a "lab" for testing my earliest, somewhat clumsy, attempts at praying for the sick. Thank you, Metroplex Chapel.

Skyline Wesleyan Church, a congregation in the suburbs of San Diego where I have served since 1995, has continued to receive my teaching on healing. One of my greatest joys has been to witness the healings that have come as I have prayed—briefly and simply—over any ill person leaving the weekend services. These times of prayer have been some of my most joyous moments both in expectant faith in God and in the privilege of being a "hands-on" pastor. I pray most expectantly for healing—and see the greatest results—in that rather unspectacular setting, the doorway of the church. I love being with you, Skyline Church family.

From 1983 to 1987, I experienced an explosive "love affair" with Jesus from which I have never recovered. During that time, God did not permit me to read any book from my substantial library. I read only the Bible. Thursday fast days were filled with insights from Scripture that I had never seen before. I learned spiritually at a pace I'd never experienced before—and that has never been matched since. That four year period laid the foundation for my understanding of numerous spiritual topics, including healing. Although I have immensely enjoyed walking with God from the age of nine and continue to be overwhelmingly excited about my personal relationship with Christ, the period from 1983 to 1987 will always remain a "sacred era" in my personal journey. Much of what is found in this book comes from the Holy Spirit's teaching during those years of learning and growth in my life.

JIM GARLOW

San Diego
June 2005

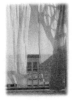

PART ONE

My Journey
into
Divine Healing

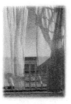

WHAT'S THE BIG DEAL ABOUT HEALING?

*Your Heavenly Father loves you and wants
you to be healthy and whole.*

"*Jim, it's Mom. They've taken your dad to the hospital . . .
I think it's pretty bad.*"

*Sunday morning services had just concluded, and two
church members, sensing the urgency of the moment, drove
Pastor Jim to Grossmont Hospital. On the way, the pastor who
had prayed so often for healing found himself at a loss for words.*

"*He's my own father,*" *Jim thought.* "*Why can't I find the
faith to believe that he'll be healed?*"

The sight in the intensive care unit was like a scene from a movie. Monitors flashed and beeped all about the room. Pastor Jim's father lay on a bed, pale, with tubes and wires seeming to be attached all over his body. Pastor Jim edged into the room, bewildered by what he saw.

"Jim, I'm so glad you're here," his mother said.

"How is he, Mom?"

"Not good, son. We need to pray."

Jim laid a hand on his dad's shoulder. Tears welled in his eyes as he choked out a brief prayer. "Oh God, help Dad. Make him well."

The blood pressure indicator suddenly plummeted. Jim got the nurse's attention and gestured anxiously toward the low number. She gave a worried look and said, "I'll have to ask you to wait outside."

Pastor Jim and his mother retreated to the waiting room, feeling confused and defeated. A few hours later they got the news.

"I'm sorry. He's gone."

I don't fully understand divine healing. I have studied it. I've learned a great deal about it. I've even experienced it. Yet I do not know all there is to know about God's healing power. So the purpose of this book is not to answer every question that could possibly be raised about the subject or to convince every skeptic in the world that God still heals. The purpose of this book is to tell what I do know about healing and to call the

—∞—

I don't fully understand divine healing, but I do know that God still heals.

church to pray more and to pray more effectively for healing. God still heals, and when God's people believe that and cry out in faith, his healing power will be released. I picture God's healing power flowing like a stream from heaven. And I'd like to see more people touched by that stream and made whole.

THE RIVER OF HEALING

I was reared in a godly home. My parents read the Bible daily and frequently shared comforting scriptures with others. Every time my father saw people traumatized or hurt, he took them to Psalm 46. In my ministry I've done the same thing. I read the opening verses of this text at nearly every bedside and funeral. They state —

> God is our refuge and strength,
>   an ever-present help in trouble.
> Therefore we will not fear, though the earth give way
>   and the mountains fall into the heart of the sea,
> though its waters roar and foam
>   and the mountains quake with their surging.

The river is a symbol of life in Hebrew literature. Psalm 46 goes on to say —

> There is a river whose streams make glad the city of God,
>   the holy place where the Most High dwells,
> God is within her, she will not fall.

Here is the truth about healing: God is a loving heavenly Father, and he wants to heal his children. The foundation of this teaching is the firm belief that God eagerly desires to give good gifts to his children.

That, finally, is why we believe that God still heals: he is a God of love, and he wants to bless us with life. So this book is an encouragement to pray. Yes, there are answers to the intellectual questions that we ask about healing. But more than that, there is encouragement to take the Father at his Word and call out to him when we are in need.

NO CONDEMNATION

Ironically, it is when we most need God's healing power that we may have the hardest time asking for it. It can be the most difficult to exercise our authority in Jesus Christ precisely when we need it most—when we are harassed by the Enemy, when we are suffering, or when we are ill. It can be difficult for us to pray for our own families. It may be hardest for us to pray for ourselves. Yet that is precisely when we most need to cry out to the Father, depending upon his mercy and asking for the good gifts that he longs to give.

Some people may experience anxiety or false guilt about the subject of healing. They might think, "If I would have known more, then so-and-so would have been healed," or, "If I had done a better job, then so-and-so wouldn't have died." I want to set your mind at ease on that subject. We will never make the subject of healing a reason for condemnation. Romans 8:1 says, "Therefore, there is now no condemnation for those who are in Christ Jesus," so if you are a believer in Jesus Christ, do not receive condemnation or guilt. What we will do is examine the Scriptures and discover how we can take advantage of the healing power that God wants to release and how we can pray effectively for the healing of others.

The story that began this chapter is mine. Several years ago I was called to the hospital on a Sunday afternoon. My father had been hospitalized for what I later learned would be the final moments of his life. As I entered the hospital, I was intimidated by what I saw. Dad was in the intensive care unit, and the room was filled with tubes, monitors, wires, and medical equipment. Medical staff members were rushing around to provide care to him. The whole situation was very stressful. It was a difficult place in which to pray for healing. I prayed, yet I felt very defeated by the experience. My dad passed away at 5:00 p.m. that day.

After that experience, I had two options. I could have blamed myself for not praying more effectively for healing. I could have said something like, "If I would have exercised the authority that I should have, my dad would be alive today." Or I could have made another choice, which is what I did, to feel the affirmation of my heavenly Father, and say to myself, "I will do my best to continue praying for healing and to learn what it takes to be more effective in this ministry."

> No one should feel guilt about being ill or about praying for healing. This teaching is not a basis for condemnation.

During the course of writing this book, Carol and I have prayed for many people. We have been encouraged by seeing people healed. At the same time, we know the disappointment of praying for the sick and watching as their condition continues to deteriorate. In fact, a friend who worked with us to develop this manuscript is in his thirtieth year of suffering from a serious chronic illness. Yet we continue to pray for the sick. Why? Because God has said to do it.

God is longing to release his healing power to his children. He wants us to be made whole. As we begin to take him at his Word, believing that he does still heal, and begin to pray for healing, we will enter the stream of his power and experience greater health and wholeness. The purpose of this book is to motivate the church to believe that

God heals and to pray consistently and effectively for healing.

When that happens, the deaf will hear, the lame will walk, and God's will is done on earth, just as it is in heaven.

LET'S PRAY

Father—

I admit that this subject makes me uneasy. I believe that you can do mighty miracles, but I find it hard to accept the thought that you will heal me. I have been frustrated by my inability to pray and by the lack of results when I have prayed. I come to you now, Lord, in faith. I believe that you love me, and I ask you to lead me into truth.

Thank you, Father.

Amen.

For small group discussion questions on this chapter and additional resources on healing, visit www.wesleyan.org/gsh.

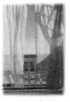

DO WE HAVE TO TALK ABOUT THIS?

Healing matters to God, so it should matter to us.

"Here we go again," Karl muttered as the pastor announced his preaching text. "Another inspired word from woo-woo Williams."

Karl's wife, Jenny, shushed him with a not-so-gentle poke in the ribs.

Pastor Williams was in the middle of a six-part series of messages titled Experiencing God's Power. Last week's message was "Deliverance: The Power to Overcome." Karl was *interested at first because he was trying to quit smoking. A little divine help couldn't hurt. But his interest faded when the pastor talked about being filled with the Holy Spirit. "Sounds wacko to me," Karl said later.*

This week's topic was divine healing. Karl listened with growing distaste as the pastor recounted miracles from the Bible and claimed that God still heals people supernaturally. Karl's mind was flooded with images of TV preachers telling people to place one hand on the television and pray to "Je-uh-sus." He closed his eyes and concentrated on his golf swing.

During the ride home, Jenny asked, "So what did you think of the sermon?"

"I'd rather not talk about it," Karl said. "Where do you want to eat?"

Divine healing is a controversial subject to some. It makes some people uncomfortable. It can be difficult to talk about. The subject can arouse such strong emotions that simply raising it for discussion can put an end to a conversation. To those who have never considered the idea that God miraculously heals people, divine healing may sound bizarre or far-fetched. To others, who have prayed for healing and seen no results, the topic can be a frustrating, even painful, one. Perhaps you feel some of that tension now. You may have been mildly uncomfortable as you read the first few pages of this book without knowing why. Perhaps you wondered—

- So why do we have to talk about this?
- Isn't it enough to simply believe in Jesus?
- Can't we leave this difficult subject alone?

Those are valid questions. Why stir up painful emotions within ourselves and controversy within the body of Christ by discussing a subject that seems to raise more questions than it answers?

WHY HEALING MATTERS

How do we know that healing is an important subject? Here are five reasons to talk about this subject even though it may be uncomfortable to do so.

THE BIBLE TALKS ABOUT IT

The Bible is God's Word to us, so any subject on which the Bible speaks should command our attention. Healing is spoken of often in Scripture. Major segments of the New Testament talk about it. In fact, major sections of the books of Matthew, Mark, and Luke are devoted to this subject. Those books are often referred to as the synoptic Gospels because they offer a synopsis of the life and ministry of Jesus. That means that healing was considered one of the most important aspects of Jesus' ministry by three of the people who observed or carefully investigated it. If healing mattered that much to the people who were close to Jesus, then it should be something we take seriously.

THE FATHER CARES ABOUT IT

Here's another clue to the importance of healing—the Father is interested in it. God came up with the idea of healing. It was he who determined that the sick and diseased body needs to be made well. The Father wants his children to be whole. If that's important to him, it should be important to us as well.

JESUS IS INTERESTED IN IT

A third reason to take healing seriously is that Jesus is interested in it. Take a look at this incident in Jesus' life, recorded in Matthew 9:35–10:1.

> Jesus went through all the towns and villages, teaching in their synagogues, preaching the good news of the kingdom and healing every disease and sickness. When he saw the crowds, he had compassion on them, because they were harassed and helpless, like sheep without a shepherd. Then he said to his disciples, "The harvest is plentiful but the workers are few. Ask the Lord of the harvest, therefore, to send out workers into his harvest field."
>
> He called his twelve disciples to him and gave them authority to drive out evil spirits and to heal every disease and sickness.

You may have heard those words before. If so, it is almost certain that you heard them applied to the subject of world missions. The phrase "send out workers into his harvest field" is so universally connected to evangelism that it makes us automatically think of sending missionaries to some foreign land. But that's not what these verses are about. The call to evangelize the world is a vitally important one, but it's not the call of this passage. Notice what Jesus was doing immediately before he issued this call to his disciples. He was teaching in their synagogues, preaching the good news of the kingdom, and *healing every disease and sickness*. It is as if Jesus is saying, "There are an awful lot of sick people out there, and I'm just one person. I need to multiply the work I'm doing by inviting others to join me in it." So he called the Twelve and sent them out with authority to cast out demons and to heal the sick. The ministry of healing was extremely important to Jesus.

There are a couple of terms in this passage that we should notice. First, notice that when Jesus saw the crowds, he had *compassion* for them because they were harassed. A compassionate person always cares when people are sick. Jesus did, and we should too. A second term to note is the word *harassed*. In the original language, that word is a wrestling term. It is as if the people were pinned down to the mat and the referee was counting them out.

And like sheep without a shepherd, they were completely helpless. There simply weren't enough people to help them. Then there is the term *send out*. That is a very active, almost violent, term in the Greek language. Jesus was literally commanding his disciples to pray that the Holy Spirit would fling workers into the field. The need is great, yet the workers are few, and Jesus is greatly concerned that his followers should be active in meeting that need. Are we? Are you?

> Divine healing may be controversial—yet Jesus was not afraid to talk about it.

A second scripture passage, Luke 9:37–43, echoes the concern that Jesus has for healing. There we see that the disciples were trying to cast out demons from a young man. In this passage, it specifically states that the boy was in need of both exorcism *and* physical healing (see verse 42). But Jesus' disciples were unable to accomplish it. When Jesus heard that, he said, "O unbelieving and perverse generation, how long shall I stay with you and put up with you? Bring [the boy] here." Then Jesus healed the boy.

When Jesus said "unbelieving and perverse generation," he was talking about his own followers! That's strong language, and Jesus directed it toward his own disciples. It is as if he was saying, "C'mon, guys, get with the program! Watch how I do it, then do the same." Jesus felt intense about this boy's need for healing. You can sense his exasperation about the fact that the disciples were ineffective in meeting the need. Clearly, Jesus wants his followers to understand how to pray so that others will become well. Healing matters to Jesus.

WE NEED HEALING

Healing matters to God, and it is mentioned frequently in the Bible. But most of us don't need a history lesson to see why the subject of healing is important. We know healing matters because we know we need to be healed. It is easy enough to ignore this subject when you are well, but the moment you or a loved one walks into a doctor's office and hears the word *cancer*, you will become vitally interested in healing. At that moment, anyone of us would want to be surrounded by people of faith who know how to pray for the sick.

Even if you are not suffering illness yourself, you will undoubtedly be moved to compassion by the needs of others. Anyone who has a deep concern for others—as Jesus does—will care about their well being. Not long ago I asked the pastoral care leader in our congregation to give a daily report on the need for healing in our church. I was amazed at the volume of requests for healing prayer. And the problems mentioned were serious. On one day the report included people dealing with strokes, knee replacements, heart attacks, lung transplants, heart attacks, brain tumors, prostate surgery, gall bladder surgery, knee surgery, pancreatic problems, heart bypass surgery, extended hospitalization, cancer, degenerative arthritis, brain tumors, oral surgery, esophageal surgery, sinusitis, insomnia, back surgery, internal bleeding, pneumonia, ovarian cancer, and kidney disease. That was the report for *one day* in our congregation. The need is truly staggering. All around us, people are dealing with health problems of all kinds. Some of them are close to us, our loved ones. Perhaps you yourself are dealing with a painful or life-threatening illness. Why talk about healing? Because we need healing. Healing matters to all of us because we are all affected by sickness.

Healing Is Part of the Great Battle

Healing can be a very personal subject. When we are in need of healing for ourselves, we think of little else. Yet divine healing has implications far beyond you and me and our bodies. Healing is part of the great contest between Jesus and Satan.

In much of the New Testament, particularly in Matthew, Mark, and Luke, many of the terms that are used have distinctly militaristic overtones. The Bible portrays a cosmic struggle between good and evil. One side is going to win, and the other side is going to lose. John Wimber taught that this battle is now raging on five distinct fronts:

- Evangelism—the battle for the human heart.
- Healing—the battle for the human body.
- Deliverance—the battle for the human emotions. In a sense, this front also involves the body because its implications are played out in our actions.
- Nature—the battle for the physical world, of which we see some clues such as Jesus' calming of the Sea of Galilee.
- Death—the battle for our ultimate destiny, won by Jesus through his resurrection.

These are the five arenas in which the contest between Jesus and Satan is played out, and we are involved in that contest! Jesus fought against the power of darkness by healing those who suffered disease, and we ought to do the same. That is made clear by a reading of Luke and Acts. These New Testament books are really one narrative in two parts, written by the same author. As you read the book of Luke, you see the healing ministry of Jesus. Everywhere he went, Jesus cast out demons, preached the good news, and healed the sick. Then Jesus went to heaven, giving his disciples a commission to carry on his work. And what did they do? The book of Acts gives the record of their ministry. The apostles carried on that same preaching and healing ministry wherever they went. Theirs was a ministry of evangelism, healing, and deliverance.

Now it is up to us. The task of the church is to carry on the ministry of Jesus. Whatever Jesus did, we need to be doing. What did Jesus do? He cast out demons, preached the good news, and *healed the sick*. The church today has concentrated a good deal of effort on evangelism, and rightly so. I'm happy to see that many churches across the nation are growing. We are making converts.

> Jesus was deeply moved by the plight of sick people and called us to share his compassion. If he prayed for the sick, shouldn't we?

But are we healing the sick? Have we neglected an important part of the Master's mission? Are we as concerned about redeeming the body as we are the soul? There is a cosmic battle now taking place, and that battle involves the physical world. Our Lord has won that battle, triumphing over his Enemy at the empty tomb. We can participate in that victory by extending his healing power to those who are in need.

THE GOAL

It's important that we take healing seriously. We need to talk about this subject and understand what Scripture says about it. Yet understanding healing is not our goal. We want to know what the Bible says, but even knowledge is not, ultimately, what counts. What really matters is that God's healing power is released in our lives with the result that people are made well. My goal in writing this book— and, I hope, your goal after reading it—is to pray more effectively so that people will be healed. We want to see God's power at work;

therefore, we are willing to stretch ourselves by talking about a subject that has been maligned and misunderstood within the church.

So it's time to have this conversation. It's time to talk about healing, to understand it, and—most of all—to pray for it. The need is great, but the workers are few. Will you join me in this vital work of Jesus Christ, the ministry of divine healing?

LET'S PRAY

Father—

I pray that you will stir up a concern within your church for those who suffer. Let us have the same compassion for others that we see in our Lord Jesus Christ. Through your Holy Spirit, I pray that you will speak to me now, leading me to see the suffering of others and to care deeply about them. Impress me again, Father, with your love, and make me willing to love others as you love me.

In Jesus' name I ask this.

Amen.

For small group discussion questions on this chapter and additional resources on healing, visit www.wesleyan.org/gsh.

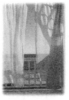

THREE

Am I the Only One Who Finds This Hard to Believe?

To accept divine healing requires a step of faith.

Rachel loved meeting with the girls in her Bible study group, all women about her age, all with kids in preschool. Tuesday mornings were a haven of grownup conversation and guilt-free croissants.

But lately Rachel found the gatherings a bit uncomfortable. Although she'd grown up in church and been a Christian nearly all her life, she was beginning to question some of the things she'd always taken for granted.

Becky, who led the informal Bible studies, seemed so sure about everything. Right and wrong were always black-and-white to her. She was even more dogmatic about her belief in miracles. Every week, the group prayed over a laundry list of great aunts and grandmothers who suffered everything from gout to Alzheimer's disease. Nobody ever got better, but Becky soldiered on, calling the group to expect a miracle every time.

Becky asked for prayer requests, and several of the women mentioned ailing relatives. Rachel sat silently, staring at the tablecloth. "What's wrong with me?" she wondered. "Am I the only one who finds this hard to believe?"

I didn't always believe that God heals people. I knew that he *could* heal, but I didn't have any evidence that he still did. That may sound surprising, given the fact that I literally grew up in church and was called to pastoral ministry at a very young age. I had been taught the Scriptures as a child and believed in God with my whole heart. But I had trouble believing that people could be supernaturally healed. I wanted to have great faith, but it seemed that I had only doubts. My journey to accept divine healing unfolded over several years. That journey began in the late 1970s in the city of Trenton, New Jersey, where I served a tiny congregation as student pastor.

QUESTIONS AND DOUBTS

Fourteen people attended First Wesleyan Church on my first Sunday there. It wasn't a big church, but it was my first pastorate, and I was working on a doctorate at Drew University in Madison, New Jersey, and was eager to apply my classroom knowledge to real life among these good people. I got that chance before church one Sunday when a lady named Mrs. Bailey came to me and said, "Pastor, I'm sick, and I need you to pray for me."

I froze. I knew virtually nothing about praying for healing, and the blank look on my face must have said so because Mrs. Bailey continued, "The Bible does say to come to the elders and ask for prayer, doesn't it?"

For the life of me, I could not remember where that passage was located, but I said, "Yes, it does."

"Well," she said, "You're an elder, and I'm coming to be anointed with oil."

Believe me, at twenty-eight years of age, I certainly didn't feel like an elder. On top of that, I don't recall that I had ever seen someone anointed with oil before that time. I had grown up in a wonderful Christian home and had attended a great church, but we didn't pray for the sick very much at all. By this time I held three master's degrees—one in New Testament studies, one in divinity, and one in theology and church history—and I was completing doctoral studies in church history, but I still had no idea what she meant when she asked to be anointed with oil. It sounds hilarious now, but all I could think of was a can of motor oil! I needed to stall for time, so I asked Mrs. Bailey to meet me in another part of the church a bit later.

Meanwhile, I went to find a godly woman named Irma Weaver. Irma was about seventy-three years old and had previously served as pastor of this congregation for about ten years. I found her sitting in the sanctuary and raced over to her. "Mrs. Weaver," I said, "we're going to need you downstairs, please. We'd like to anoint Mrs. Bailey with oil." She seemed to know exactly what I was talking about, so I just kept going. "Mrs. Weaver, out of deference to you, I'd like for you to be the one to anoint Mrs. Bailey." To my great relief, she said she would.

As we walked downstairs, I wondered what this was going to look like. Would she pour oil all over Mrs. Bailey? Would she use a whole quart? Would we need a tarp for the floor? What actually happened was that Mrs. Weaver took a small vial of clear oil, dabbed a drop onto her finger, and placed it on Mrs. Bailey's forehead. Then she prayed for her. That was all. Looking back, I recall that as a wonderful, spiritual moment. But at the time, I admit, it seemed a little spooky.

A SERIES OF FAILURES

The years passed. I finished my degree and eventually accepted the pastorate of a church in the heart of the Dallas–Ft. Worth area. It was 1983. That was the year of what I call "the explosion" in my life. That year marked a renewal of my love affair with Jesus. It began with a stirring in my heart, a hunger to know Jesus and to know his power. I wanted to understand what he was like. I wanted to get past all the theological talk and truly know the Jesus who is all-powerful, who can change people and rearrange lives—who heals the sick. So I began reading Scripture and studying as aggressively as I could. I also began praying for the sick. Starting in March of that year, I prayed for every sick person I came around. I was truly dedicated. For a span of six months, nearly every person I prayed for got *sicker*. I began to imagine that sick people were running away from me. One person jokingly said, "Jim, so-and-so is in the hospital, but please don't come—we know you'll pray them straight through the Pearly Gates!" The results from my prayer were terrible, and I became very discouraged.

Then one day a lady named Willadene said, "Jim, will you come to the hospital? My dad is there."

I wanted to say, "Lady, with my track record, you don't want me anywhere near the place!" But I knew that she desperately wanted someone to pray for her father, so I agreed to go.

I wasn't prepared for what I saw when I entered that hospital room. Willadene's father appeared to be in his nineties. His teeth were gone, his body was shriveled, and there seemed to be tubes attached to him everywhere. "Oh no," I thought. "This guy doesn't stand a chance with me even standing in the room, let alone praying for him." All I could think of was the string of failures I'd had for the last six months.

I turned to Willadene and asked, "How do you want me to pray?"

She said, "You know, Jim, just pray that he will go on home to be with the Lord."

I thought, "Yes! This is my specialty, my gift to the body of Christ!" I felt my faith surging right through the roof, so I prayed, "Oh Lord, take this brother home!" I honestly thought the man would die right then and there—everybody else had. But as I opened my eyes, I saw that he was staring right back at me.

> My own journey to accept this teaching included many questions, doubts, and failures.

Back then I thought authority in prayer was directly proportional to sound volume, so I simply prayed louder. I really cranked it up and hollered, "OH GOD, YOU REMEMBER WHAT A GOOD SUNDAY SCHOOL TEACHER THIS MAN WAS." I thought my recommendation might encourage God to let the man into heaven. But when I opened my eyes again, the fellow was still there, looking right at me. "What do I have to do," I wondered, "cut off his oxygen?" I was dumbfounded that the man was still alive. Finally, I left the room and said to Willadene, "When something happens, call me."

The next morning at 7:00, the phone rang and it was Willadene. As soon as I heard her voice, I started thinking about funeral preparations. But she said, "Jim, you won't believe what happened. My dad sat up in bed and called me by name!"

I was really ticked. I thought, "God, what is the deal here? One of us isn't holding up his end of the bargain—and it isn't me!" It had been six months since I began to pray for healing, and almost everyone I'd prayed for had gotten sicker. But the one time I *tried* to pray someone into heaven, he wouldn't go. As odd as it sounds, I was discouraged because this man's condition had improved. I was ready to give up healing altogether.

THE POWER OF GOD

The very next morning, I attended a breakfast meeting with a group of pastors. I purposely arrived late because I knew the agenda for the meeting. We were going to discuss a number of items that had nothing to do with the concerns I was facing in my ministry. I had no interest in the meeting; all I could think about was healing.

I took my place at the end of a long, narrow table with nineteen other pastors. I intended to stay for the meal, then quietly slip out when the discussion began. I was just about to make my fast break when a pastor named Jack Smith announced, "I've brought a song evangelist with me. This man has traveled all over the country providing music for church services and revival meetings, but he's sick. He has a respiratory condition, and he can barely sing. He's so ill that he can't even drive from city to city. On some nights, he's so ill that he can't sing at all. So before we talk about the agenda items, we need to pray for his healing." Then Jack said the very last thing I wanted to hear. He turned to me and said, "Hey, Jim, you know all about healing. Why don't you pray for him?" At that moment, all nineteen pastors turned to look at me.

You've heard about those "arrow prayers" that people shoot up to heaven in an emergency? Well I prayed one. I said, "Lord, I don't think that's one bit funny!" But I knew that I had to pray for the man—and I wanted to. So I stepped over to where he was seated and laid my left hand on his shoulder and my right hand on his chest. I have no idea why I prayed the words I did, because I'd never prayed this way before. In a strong voice and with great authority I said, "In the name of Jesus, I command you to come out of him!"

Even as I said the words, I knew they sounded like a poor imitation of a televangelist. "Oops," I thought. "Did I really say that?" I had no idea what to do next.

Immediately the man started rocking back and forth, and I felt a sensation in my hand that I had never felt before. It felt like ripples of skin coming up in my right hand. I had never experienced anything like it before and never have since. Meanwhile, the man continued rocking back and forth. Now I began to get worried. "Oh no!" I thought. "I've killed him right here in front of all these people." Just then, the man gasped and looked straight up at me. He claimed, "Something came out of me."

Since I was standing in front of all those pastors, I didn't want to appear too surprised. I tried to act as if this happened all the time when I prayed. "Well guys," I said casually, "sometimes it just happens that way." In reality, I didn't have the foggiest idea what was going on. But one thing was certain—the man was healed. He felt better immediately and was able to breathe freely for the first time in months. Everyone was amazed at what had taken place.

Then they all lined up in front of me! '

"Pray for me too," said a pastor named Bill.

"OK, Bill," I said, trying to sound confident. "What's your problem?"

"Hemorrhoids," he said.

I wanted to say, "But Bill, I'm not a hemorrhoid man! I'm a respiratory man. Can't you tell?" But with nineteen guys watching me,

I had to do something. So I said, "Bill, I'll pray for you, but maybe we can dispense with the laying on of hands." It was a comical scene, but I did pray for the man and he was healed instantly. I've kept in contact with him over the years, and he has reported that his healing was complete. So now I had healed one wheezing song evangelist and one guy with hemorrhoids.

Regardless of where you are in your journey, you can pray for the sick.

The next pastor in line said, "There's a ringing in my ears. It's been there for years. I can barely hear, and sometimes it's hard to preach. Both my dad and brother have it too." I prayed for him, and he was healed. After that, many more came. Within a few minutes, we all sensed that something important was taking place. It wasn't just that people were being healed; it was that God was there, and everyone knew it. What happened next was truly amazing.

One pastor stood up and addressed another. He said, "Your church is only about a mile from mine, and you and I have been competitors. I want to ask your forgiveness for that. I know that your church has been suffering financially, and we'd like to send some of our offerings to help you out."

Then a pastor named Terri who had just lost about one hundred pounds rose and said "You've all been complimenting me on how much weight I've lost, but I haven't told you guys that one day I was crying out to God and somebody laid hands on me. I was set free from a spirit, and that's how it happened. I never had the courage to tell you what happened."

Mark, another pastor, stood up and said, "I want to ask forgiveness from all of you for the spirit of jealousy I've had. Will you forgive me?" We all cried together as he confessed.

Two hours later, we left that meeting never having talked about the items on the agenda. But we experienced genuine revival, and that happened, I believe, because we were willing to trust God in the area of divine healing. That day was the turning point in my journey to embrace this marvelous teaching. That day marked the beginning of a healing ministry in my life as the power of God was displayed among us.

YOUR JOURNEY

We are all at different points on the journey of faith. Perhaps you have unanswered questions about the idea of divine healing. You may be skeptical about it, just as I was. Merely reading this book may be one step on your journey to trust God fully in this area. Let me challenge you to do one thing. I encourage you to go beyond thinking about healing or even studying Scripture but to begin praying for the sick. It is true that there is a natural and right time to go and be with the Lord. There's an appointed time for that for each one of us. You will experience times, as I did, when those for whom you pray are not healed and may even die. Yet I am so glad that I did not give up on the idea that God heals. I was tempted to do just that. I was nearly ready to believe that no person I prayed for would ever be healed. Thankfully, I persevered in prayer.

You can do the same. Regardless of your questions or where you are in your journey, you can pray for the sick. You can learn to minister to others in the arena of healing. God is not looking for superstars or healing geniuses. He's looking for a band of people through whom he can release his power.

Could you be one of them?

LET'S PRAY

Father—

Help me to trust you. Give me the faith to take you at your word and believe that you are all powerful. Please be patient with me when I am doubtful, and strengthen my faith. I want to experience all that you have for me. Make me ready to receive all that you are willing to give.

In Jesus' name I pray.

Amen.

For small group discussion questions on this chapter and additional resources on healing, visit www.wesleyan.org/gsh.

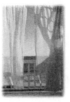

WHY IS HEALING SO MISUNDERSTOOD?

Although this practice has sometimes been abused,
healing is still God's plan for his children.

"Mom, what's this check for?"

Valerie Lucas visited her aging mother nearly every day, but it had been a couple of months since she had helped her pay bills. While balancing her mother's checkbook, Valerie noticed a payment for one thousand dollars to The Apostolic Faith Center, Inc.

Charlotte Evans said nothing, staring intently at the television screen.

"Mom," Valerie became insistent. "A thousand dollars is a lot of money. Is this a church or something?"

"Oh, that," Charlotte said absently. "That's for my miracle."

"She's got to be kidding," Valerie thought, "there's no way my mother could be that foolish." Valerie stepped between her mother and the television set, tuned to a religious station.

"Mom, you didn't send money to that TV preacher, did you?"

"Well, I think I sent a little," Charlotte said hesitantly. "My arthritis has been so bad. And Pastor Milton knew all about it. He prayed for me, for my miracle. . . ."

Valerie didn't know whether to laugh or cry. She flipped through the check register and found two more payments to the televangelist's ministry, one for five hundred dollars, the other for two thousand. Her face went white with anger. "I can't believe it," she said aloud. "My own mother, taken in by this healing nonsense."

D ivine healing is one of the most misunderstood teachings in some churches. Mention the words *miracle* or *faith healing* in some congregations, and you're likely to be met with skepticism—or worse. Some Christians genuinely believe that divine healing is a sham, a ruse played upon those who are naïve or overly trusting. Others are simply wary of anything that seems too good to be true. Either way, a discussion of this powerful truth may be answered with anything from an amused smile to active criticism.

Why is healing so misunderstood? If divine healing really is God's plan for his people, why wouldn't all believers embrace it?

What accounts for the apathy, skepticism, and even criticism that is often leveled at this teaching? There are two reasons why divine healing is misunderstood and sometimes maligned.

POOR MODELS

When you hear the words *faith healing*, you probably think of the various TV preachers you've seen over the years. I've seen them too, and I have to admit that some of them—but by no means all—were rather strange. Years ago when I would watch some of these preachers, I didn't know whether to be entertained or upset. Everything about them seemed comical. Even the way they spoke sounded funny to me, always seeming to mispronounce words. They would heal in *JE-uh-sus'* name and then shout *Gu-LO-ree!* To be honest, I was completely turned off by them—and the teaching they seemed to espouse. I wanted no part of it.

Then several years ago, a friend of mine came for a visit. He had done an enormous amount of research on healing. He and his team had examined reports of healing in a microscopic way. They had looked at doctors' reports, witness testimonies, and even X-rays to determine whether the accounts were genuine. They had spent about five years on the project.

Poor role models have discouraged many from believing that God still heals.

Since my friend had done so much research on the subject, I decided to ask him about a particular TV preacher that I'd seen. This preacher seemed so strange to me that I wouldn't have wanted him living in my neighborhood, let alone praying for my healing. I used to poke fun at the way he talked and some of the odd mannerisms that he had when praying for healing. So I asked my friend, "What about this preacher—is he for real?" I fully expected him to say that the man was a fraud, but he did not.

"Oh yes," my friend replied, "he's genuine. We interviewed several of the people he's prayed for. We even interviewed some of the medical people who treated them. Time after time, we found that reports were authentic."

I was shocked. "How do you explain that?" I asked my friend. "This guy looks to me as if he should be locked up!"

I'll never forget my friend's reply. He said, "Healing is so controversial and so many people feel that it's beneath their dignity that most people want nothing to do with it. I'm convinced that's the reason God works through the kind of people you're seeing on television. He uses people who are willing to be misunderstood and criticized yet move forward."

That response sobered and quieted me. From that moment on, I stopped criticizing. I shouldn't have been criticizing that preacher in the first place, and I have never done it since. I prayed, "Oh, God, have I become so sophisticated that I won't allow myself to be misunderstood in doing your work?" From that day forward, I resolved to pursue God's will in the area of healing even if other people thought I was odd for doing so.

Certainly there have been frauds in the area of healing. And certainly there have been poor models in this area. Not all of the people who practice faith healing are people we would want to emulate. But we must never allow these poor models to discourage us from accepting the wonderful truth that God wants his children to be well.

POOR TEACHING

A second reason the doctrine of divine healing is misunderstood is that it has sometimes been poorly taught. Not all faith healers are good role models, and not all teaching on the subject of healing is valid. Let's examine the four fundamental views about healing.

Denial. The first view is not very popular, but some people do hold it. This view states that miraculous healing never happened. During the mid-twentieth century, a German theologian named Rudolph Bultmann taught a theory of Bible interpretation called *demythologization*. That theory holds that the Bible is filled with myths, which should not be taken as factual. Bultmann interpreted all miracle stories that way and believed they were useful only for their spiritual lessons. He would have said, for example, that if the Bible says that Jesus restored someone's sight, it does not mean that Jesus healed that person physically. What the Bible is trying to communicate is that Jesus gave that person new understanding, not the literal ability to see.

Bultmann's teaching spread to America where it is taught in some leading seminaries. As a result, there are people who believe that divine healing never happened, not even in Bible times. They simply do away with the possibility of miracles, even the resurrection of Christ, claiming that such things never happened—and never will.

Historical. A second school of thought with regard to divine healing is that it happened at one time but doesn't happen now. People who hold this view would admit that Jesus and others performed miracles during Bible times. They believe, however, that the age of miracles ended at the close of the New Testament period, about A.D. 100. Since that time, there have been no miracles.

Occasional. A third view is that divine healing happens but only occasionally. Some people believe that while miracles can happen, they are extremely rare. People who hold this view tend to pray this way: "Father please heal so-and-so *if it is your will*." They condition all of their prayers on the idea that God may not be inclined to heal in any given case.

It is not a bad thing to pray for the will of God to be accomplished. Jesus taught us to pray in just that way. That's the way he prayed, and we want to follow his example. But when Jesus healed, he never said, "Be healed—*if* it's the will of the Father." He always regarded healing to be the Father's desire.

I used to subscribe to this third view. Then several years ago, I began to study healing. Until that time I had always prayed for healing using the words "if it is your will" or something similar. But after I studied the matter, I stopped using that phrase when praying for healing because Jesus never prayed that way about healing. Jesus never even hinted that the Father might not want a person to be well. Jesus knew that the Father *always* wants people to be well, so if they continue to be ill, there must be another reason.

> Most people begin this journey with some apprehension. It takes faith to overcome that fear and trust God.

Why is it that the phrase "if it is your will" is so often used by Christians when praying for healing? I think it is because our prayers for healing have been ineffective and we feel the need to cover ourselves. We pray that way so that we can later say, "It must not have been God's will for that person to be healed." But there is a better way to understand God's will for healing.

Normal. The fourth view of healing is that it *is* the Father's will for people to be well, so healing is the normal result of prayer. Let's explore this idea further. When children get sick, their parents want them to get well. We would never say to a parent, "I hope your child gets well, if that's what you really want." All good parents want their children to be well. There are many good earthly fathers, but our Heavenly Father is better than any of us. Can you imagine God saying to himself, "I think I'd like for my child to be ill for just a little bit longer"? It is *always* God's will for his children to be well. Divine healing is not impossible, and it is not merely occasional; it is the result of our prayer based on the Father's mercy.

Right now you are probably asking, "If God wants people to be well, then why is anyone sick? If healing is normal, then why doesn't it always happen?" Those are good questions, and we'll explore them later in this book. For now, however, the important thing is to realize that God is a good Heavenly Father and does want his children to be well.

Overcoming Fear

Second Timothy 1:7 says God has not given us a spirit of timidity, but a spirit of power, of love, and of self-discipline. Many people are timid, even fearful, of the doctrine of divine healing. Frankly, some have good reason to be. This teaching may have been abused more than any other teaching in the church. Some unscrupulous characters have done great damage by misapplying this teaching.

Yet healing is real. And our Heavenly Father wants us to seize it boldly and apply it to our lives. He does not want us to live in fear but to enjoy the power that he is willing to release through his Holy Spirit. God's healing power can be released in the world through our prayers — through *your* prayers — if we will have faith and courage enough to ignore the skeptics, disregard the critics, and take the Father at his word.

Let's Pray

Father —

I believe that you are a loving God, yet I am uneasy about this teaching. I don't want to miss your blessing, but I don't want to be duped by imposters either. Give me courage, Father, and give me faith. Enable me to ignore distracting voices and to hear yours alone. Help me know your Word in the area of healing and to apply it to my life.

In Jesus' name I pray,

Amen.

For small group discussion questions on this chapter and additional resources on healing, visit www.wesleyan.org/gsh.

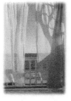

PART TWO

WHAT THE BIBLE SAYS ABOUT HEALING

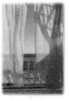

FIVE

WASN'T HEALING ONLY FOR THE EARLY CHURCH?

*Healing is an evidence of God's presence
in every place and time.*

Colleen enjoyed the citywide luncheon for Christian women as an opportunity to make Christian friends outside her own denomination. Nearly every month she met someone from a different tradition and was always amazed at how much they had in common.

During the prayer time, the leader asked people seated at each table to share prayer requests, then pray for one another. Gail, who was new to the group, told her tablemates about the struggle of dealing with her diabetic husband.

"Let's pray for Gail's husband," Colleen urged the group, "that God will heal him of this illness."

Gail returned a blank stare. "Just pray that he'll give me the grace to cope with all of this," she said.

"Of course," Colleen said, "But we'll pray for his healing too."

This time Gail was more insistent. "God's not going to heal my husband," she said flatly. "God doesn't do that sort of thing anymore; my pastor even said so. And I'm not going to give anyone false hope by pretending that he does."

S ome people object to the idea that God still heals because they believe that miraculous healing was a work that God did for a limited time, just the period recorded in the Bible. Their theory goes something like this: When the early church was just being established, God needed to "prop it up" to help keep it going. Because people in those days needed lots of courage, God gave them plenty of miraculous signs and wonders to boost their faith. Those miraculous signs included healing. But, the theory continues, God abruptly stopped performing signs and wonders once the young church was established. So you and I can't expect to see miraculous healing in our day. That was for a previous time—a previous *dispensation*—and God simply doesn't do that anymore.

FOOTPRINTS OF THE HOLY SPIRIT

The problem with that view is that it has no clear support in Scripture. It is a mistake to conclude that God simply turned off the healing spigot. There is no statement in Scripture to that effect. In fact, the Bible presents a completely contrary view of healing. According to Scripture, healing is a clear evidence of God's work. So whenever God is working—then or now—miraculous healing will be the result. Divine healing was not reserved for one time in history. It is an evidence of God's work, and we can expect to see that evidence wherever and whenever God is present including right here, right now.

HEALING PROMISED IN THE OLD TESTAMENT

Let's review what the Bible says about healing, beginning with the Old Testament. God's desire to bring healing predates the early church. This is one evidence that God intends to heal at all times. Psalm 103:1–5 says—

> Praise the Lord, O my soul;
>> all my inmost being, praise his holy name.
> Praise the Lord, O my soul,
>> and forget not all his benefits—
> who forgives all your sins
>> and heals all your diseases,
> who redeems your life from the pit
>> and crowns you with love and compassion,
> who satisfies your desires with good things
>> so that your youth is renewed like the eagle's.

This psalm was written several hundred years before the New Testament era, long before the baby church supposedly needed signs and wonders to bolster its faith. And this passage specifically states that healing is a work that God does for his children. It is a benefit, if you will, of salvation.

If I were to ask you about your work, I might inquire about the benefits you have as an employee at your company. You would know what those benefits are because they are very important. You might list such things as health insurance, sick time, and vacation pay. If your employer cut your benefits and your boss simply announced one day that the company would no longer provide benefits such as health insurance, you'd be very upset. And your employer certainly would never do something like that without informing you. Can you imagine going to the doctor one day and having the doctor's staff say, "I'm sorry, but your health insurance is no longer valid"? Healing is a good thing—a "benefit"— that God provides for his children, and it makes no sense to think that God would simply stop providing it, especially without any mention. If God were going to stop healing, he would make a very clear statement about it in Scripture. Yet there is none.

Long before the New Testament period, God stated that healing is one of the good things that he does for us. It's a benefit of our relationship with him, and that benefit is still in effect. God still heals.

JESUS' HEALING MINISTRY BEGINS

The occasion of Jesus' first sermon is recorded for us in Luke 4. The setting is Jesus' hometown of Nazareth, a very small community in the region of Galilee. Nazareth was an inauspicious place, and the place where Jesus lived was probably lowly as well. Some believe Jesus was reared by his mother, Mary, and his earthly father, Joseph, in a type of cave dug into the side of a hill. Jesus came from rather humble circumstances. It was in Nazareth that Jesus launched his ministry. It was there that he preached his first sermon, with disastrous results.

The problem arose when Jesus read from Isaiah. Seven hundred years before Jesus' time, Isaiah had announced that the Messiah would come. Jesus aroused anger in the crowd that day by claiming to be that Messiah. But what we are noting here is the role that the promised Messiah would play. Luke 4:18–19 records the words of Jesus that day. He said, "The Spirit of the Lord is on me, because he has anointed me to preach good news to the poor. He has sent me to proclaim freedom for the prisoners and recovery of sight for the blind, to release the oppressed, to proclaim the year of the Lord's favor." Notice two things: First, part of the ministry that Jesus claimed for himself as Messiah involved healing. Second, Jesus made no mention of the idea that his healing ministry would be for a limited time. Remember that Jesus spoke these words sometime around A.D. 30 and that the period of the early church extended to about A.D. 100. That's about seventy years. Nowhere does Jesus give the slightest hint that a healing ministry would last only seven decades.

Jesus specifically stated that healing was to be part of his ministry as the Messiah. Jesus launched that ministry and equipped others to join him in it. What reason is there to believe that healing should not accompany the ministry of Christ even today?

JESUS' MINISTRY CONTINUES

Let's continue looking at the healing ministry of Jesus. Matthew 9:35–10:1states: "Jesus went through all the towns and villages, teaching in their synagogues, preaching the good news of the kingdom and healing every disease and sickness." Sometimes small words carry significant meaning, and that's true in this passage. Notice that Jesus healed *every* disease and sickness. The text doesn't say that Jesus healed a *few* diseases or *some* disease. He healed every one of them. Whether it was cancer or merely a cold, Jesus healed those who needed to be made well.

Matthew 9:36–38 continues: "When he saw the crowds, he had compassion on them, because they were harassed and helpless, like sheep without a shepherd. Then he said to his disciples, 'The harvest is plentiful but the workers are few. Ask the Lord of the harvest, therefore, to send out workers into his harvest field.'" Jesus was concerned about sick people—so concerned that he called his followers to share that burden. And remember that there were no chapter and verse divisions in the original text of the Bible. Those were not added until the Middle Ages. So in this passage, the account continues right on into the next chapter. Matthew 10:1 says, "He called his twelve disciples to him and gave them authority to drive out evil spirits and to heal every disease and sickness." Here Jesus begins to *multiply* his ministry of healing. He now invites others to join the healing ministry that he announced in his very first sermon. Jesus appointed twelve Christians—"little Christs," as Martin Luther would later say—to join him in the work of healing others.

HEALING AND THE KINGDOM OF GOD

In Matthew 9:35 we see the phrase "preaching the good news of the kingdom." The Kingdom, of course, is the kingdom of heaven (also called the kingdom of God), which Jesus initiated through his ministry.

> The ministry of Jesus was saturated with healing.

That Kingdom today comprises all people who believe in Jesus, who are born again. Many people live in countries that are nominally Christian, and there are many people who are associated with a church but who have never truly been born again. So the Kingdom is not all people who would identify themselves on a survey as being Christian; it is all of the people who truly believe in Christ.

The Kingdom will have its fulfillment in heaven. But for now, the church gives the world a taste of that Kingdom—sort of like an hors d'oeuvre. The church is not the main course. It simply sets the stage for the ultimate expression of God's Kingdom. There will come a day when the reign of God is established over everything. I love the way this truth is expressed in Philippians 2:9–11. There will come a day when every knee will bow and every tongue confess the lordship of Jesus Christ. Whether they have chosen Christ as their Lord during this lifetime or not, all people will *someday* acknowledge that he is Lord over all creation. There are several views on how and when that will happen. Some believe that the church will proclaim the gospel with greater and greater authority until it dominates the entire world. Others believe that quite the reverse is true, that the world will become worse and worse until Jesus returns to establish the Kingdom by force. But either way, the present role of the church is the same. It gives the world a glimpse of what that coming Kingdom will be like.

When Jesus sent his disciples out and told them to preach "the good news of the kingdom," he was telling them to announce that this Kingdom was on its way and to offer a taste of what it would be like. It is significant that Jesus commissioned them to heal as a part of this ministry. Their foretaste of the Kingdom included healing. That gives us the very clear picture that the kingdom of God includes healing. When God establishes his full authority over an area, people are healed. The kingdom of heaven includes healing, and those who proclaim the Kingdom will be carriers of that healing power.

Is the kingdom of heaven a future concept or has it arrived? Its fulfillment will take place in the future. But the kingdom of heaven exists both "here and now" (on earth) and "there and then" (in heaven). Jesus initiated that Kingdom with his earthly ministry. Every person whose heart has come under the lordship of Jesus Christ is a member of that Kingdom. The Kingdom is here and now. Because that is true, we can experience God's healing power today just as people did in the early church. Admittedly, we will experience that power fully when the kingdom of heaven is finally made complete. Yet the Kingdom is here and now. And God still heals as part of that kingdom.

HEALING AND THE HOLY SPIRIT

Let's fast-forward to the book of Acts. As the book of Acts opens, Jesus ascends into heaven. But before he does, Jesus transfers authority to his disciples. "You will receive power," he told them, "when the Holy Spirit comes on you" (Acts 1:8). Just prior to this time, Jesus announced the Great Commission to the disciples, sending them into the world to carry on his ministry. And what follows in the book of Acts is the record of them doing exactly that. When the Holy Spirit came on the day of Pentecost, the church was born. From that day forward, Christ's followers went boldly into the world, continuing the ministry of evangelism, healing, and deliverance that Jesus had announced in his first public sermon. Not surprisingly, the record of the apostles' work is riddled with accounts of healing. Acts 2:43 reports that many wonders and miraculous signs were done by the apostles. Peter and John healed a crippled man in the temple courts (Acts 3:1–10), and Peter later raised a woman from the dead (Acts 9:36–43).

As stated earlier, there are five types of *power encounters* recorded in Scripture. One is Jesus coming against the sickness and disease brought on by the Enemy, and that is called *healing*. The second is Jesus coming against the damage done by the Enemy to people's nervous and emotional systems, and that is called *deliverance*. A third is Jesus coming against the proclivity of the human heart to sin, and that we call *evangelism*. The fourth is Jesus coming against the power of the Enemy to cause destruction in the world. Jesus did this by displaying his mastery over the forces of nature when he stilled the storm. This is a power encounter with *nature*. And the fifth power encounter is Jesus coming against the spirit of death and raising people from the dead, that is *resurrection*. When God is at work, his power will be displayed. And that power was displayed among the apostles as they continued the ministry of Jesus—as they continued advancing the kingdom of heaven—as recorded in the book of Acts.

THE MAIN COURSE

Here is the sequence of healing revealed in Scripture. In the Old Testament God promised healing as a benefit that he would provide for his children. When Jesus came to earth, he inaugurated the kingdom of heaven by announcing a ministry of healing. He later commissioned his disciples to join him in that healing work. And before he ascended into heaven, Jesus imparted authority to them so that they could continue his mission. Finally, the Holy Spirit came on the day of Pentecost, empowering the disciples to act on Jesus' command. God never intended that miraculous healing would be for a limited time. He intends to reclaim the entire world as his Kingdom, and wherever he is at work, healing will be seen.

Does it make sense that God would discontinue healing without one word of explanation in Scripture?

What God really desires is that people would see divine healing for what it is—a prelude to the kingdom of heaven that will be fully realized someday. God wants us to see healing as the hors d'oeuvre that leads us to the main course. It should merely whet our appetite for more of him.

When Jesus first sent out the Twelve, he said to them, "As you go, preach this message: 'The kingdom of heaven is near.' Heal the sick, raise the dead, cleanse those who have leprosy, drive out demons" (Matt. 10:7–8). The kingdom of heaven and healing are inextricably linked. Wherever Christ is, there his Kingdom will be. And wherever that Kingdom exists there will be healing. It was true then. It is true today.

The Apostle Paul wrote, "For the kingdom of God is not a matter of talk but of power" (1 Cor. 4:20). We long to see the day when the whole earth is reached with the gospel of Jesus Christ. But that will never happen if we merely talk about it. If that is to become a reality, there must be a manifestation of God's power in ways that we have not seen before in our lifetime. So far, we've had only the appetizers. It's time for the main course. It's time to experience the healing power of God.

LET'S PRAY

Father—

I know that you have done great works in the past. I have heard what you did for your people in ancient times, and I know that you raised Jesus from the dead. I long to see your work renewed in this time, in my life. Let your Kingdom come, Father, and your will be done, on earth as it is in heaven.

In Jesus' name I pray,
Amen.

For small group discussion questions on this chapter and additional resources on healing, visit www.wesleyan.org/gsh.

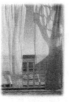

ISN'T IT ONLY IN HEAVEN THAT PEOPLE ARE TRULY HEALED?

*Wherever God's rule is fully manifested,
there is healing.*

❮❯

"I hate funeral homes," Jack Campbell thought as he entered the tiny chapel. *Mournful organ music, combined with the faint odor of disinfectant gave the place a macabre feel.*

Jack's uncle Ernie had been seventy-eight when he died after years of poor health. Jack hardly remembered his uncle except as a frail old man. Aunt Anna sat near the open casket, dressed in black. A stream of mourners made their way to her side. Jack stood in line to greet his aunt, trying to think of something to say.

"I'm sure sorry about Uncle Ernie," he offered. "He was a good man, and I know a lot of people prayed for him."

"That's kind of you, Jack," Anna replied. "I'm just glad our prayers were finally answered."

Jack was nonplussed. He stared at the corpse, then back at his aunt."

"Um, how do you mean, Aunt Anna?"

"Our prayers for healing," Anna said. "They were finally answered. Ernest is healed now, in heaven. That's what we've all been waiting for."

Jack hesitated. "Well, praise the Lord for that," he offered weakly, then squeezed Anna's hand, pretending to smile.

"I gotta get out of here," he thought, edging toward the door. "I really hate funeral homes."

One objection people have to the idea that God still heals is based on their belief that real healing occurs only in heaven. They sometimes use the term *ultimate healing* to express the idea that it is only in the next life that we will experience God's healing power. The idea is that we will experience wholeness only in our glorified state in heaven, not before. The Bible presents a different picture, however. It shows us that Jesus came to bring the kingdom of heaven to earth—at least in part. And wherever God's kingdom exists, there will be healing.

In the preceding chapter, we discovered that healing has been part of God's plan from the beginning and that it continues today. Healing isn't relegated to a particular time in the past. In this chapter, we'll see that healing isn't reserved only for an ideal time in the future. It is part of the Kingdom here and now.

Thy Kingdom Come

In Jesus' very first sermon, he announced that he was establishing a new order—the kingdom of heaven. In his hometown of Nazareth, Jesus had been invited to read Scripture at the synagogue. Here's what happened:

> He stood up to read, and the book of the prophet Isaiah was handed to him and he opened the book and found the place where it was written, "The Spirit of the Lord is on me, because he has anointed me to preach good news to the poor. He has sent me to proclaim freedom for the prisoners and recovery of sight for the blind, to release the oppressed, to proclaim the year of the Lord's favor."
>
> Then he rolled up the scroll, gave it back to the attendant and sat down. The eyes of everyone in the synagogue were fastened on him, and he began by saying to them, "Today this scripture is fulfilled in your hearing" (Luke 4:18–21).

By making that announcement, Jesus was establishing his authority. He declared the fact that he had come to establish the reign of God on earth. Not surprisingly, there was opposition to that statement. Some who were present were so offended that they even tried to kill him.

Present versus Future Age

This Scripture is an example of what is called "dualism." That simply means that there are two things happening at the same time. By reading from Isaiah, Jesus was harking back to the well-known concept of the "day of the Lord." This idea was commonly referred to by Old Testament prophets as the time when God would come to establish his reign, balance the scales, and set all things right again. Malachi said, "Surely the day is coming; it will burn like a furnace. All the arrogant and every evildoer will be stubble and that day that is coming will set them on fire, says the Lord Almighty" (Mal. 4:1). Paul picked up on this same idea in 2 Thessalonians 1:7, saying that Christ will return with blazing fire and with powerful angels, destroying the wicked. The Day of the Lord was the time when God's rule would be firmly established on earth. So when Jesus announced that Isaiah's prophecy had been fulfilled, he was saying that the Day of the Lord—the kingdom of heaven—had in fact come.

> We live in two worlds—the *already* and the *not yet.*

Obviously, however, the Kingdom has not *fully* come. We still see Satan active on earth. We are not living in heaven; we continue to occupy earth. So from the time of Jesus forward, we have lived between these two worlds—the kingdom of heaven and the kingdom of earth. Jesus came to inaugurate the Kingdom, and when he returns, it will be consummated. For now, we experience an *already* but *not yet* existence. The Kingdom has come—but it is not fully established. That is why Paul says in 1 Corinthians 10:11, "The fulfillment of the ages has come."

SIGNS OF THE KINGDOM

Jesus gave us signs of the presence of God's kingdom so that we can recognize it. One sign is a concern for the poor and downtrodden. When the rule of God is established, the disenfranchised are lifted up and protected. Another sign of the Kingdom is healing. Many people think that Jesus' healing ministry was a kind of magic act, as if he went around sprinkling fairy dust on a few lucky souls. But the healing ministry of Jesus was really an outgrowth of the Kingdom. When the reign of God is established, the power of darkness is broken. God's healing power is released, and people are made whole. That happened nearly everywhere Jesus went. When he brought the Kingdom, healing followed.

Another sign of the Kingdom is deliverance. Where God's reign is established, people are freed from the things that enslave them, including demonic affliction and addiction. Jesus came to establish God's kingdom, and that Kingdom is characterized by restoration: physical healing, deliverance from evil, and salvation.

KINGDOM SIGHTINGS

If you were to have followed Jesus after he preached that first sermon in Nazareth, you would have seen evidence of the Kingdom taking place all around him. Immediately he went out and set free a man who was demonically afflicted. Not long after that, Jesus healed Peter's mother-in-law in the city of Capernaum. He also healed a great number of others in that city. Naturally, the people were eager for Jesus to remain there, but he refused. He said, "I must preach the good news of the kingdom of God to the other towns also, because that is why I was sent" (Luke 4:43). He healed the sick, cast out demons, fed multitudes, and even raised people from the dead. When the kingdom of God comes, God's power is released. And we see that demonstrated throughout the ministry of Jesus. It is as though Jesus was delivering on a campaign promise. He had stated that the Kingdom had come, and as he went out from Nazareth, he proved that his statement was true.

CLASH OF TWO WORLDS

Before long, however, there was a clash between the two worlds—heaven and earth. As Jesus invaded the territory of

Satan, he counterattacked. On one occasion Jesus was crossing the lake with his disciples and a great storm arose, threatening to sink the boat. That was the work of the Enemy, trying to oppose the spread of God's kingdom. What did Jesus do? He stilled the storm, establishing God's peace. Shortly after that, Jesus encountered a demon-possessed man. The demon cried out to Jesus, "What do you want with me, Jesus, Son of the Most High God? I beg you, don't torture me!" (Luke 8:28). That demon had sufficient awareness to recognize that Jesus is God's son and to realize what Jesus was doing. He realized that Christ had come to reclaim his Kingdom, establishing the reign of God on earth.

Even the demonic forces recognized that there was a cataclysmic battle taking place. The kingdom of earth was being invaded by the kingdom of heaven, and sickness was a battle front in that war. Jesus said in John 10:10 that the thief had come to steal, kill, and destroy, but that he had come to bring abundant life. Jesus brought the Kingdom to earth, and with it, he brought healing.

THY WILL BE DONE

The healing work of the Kingdom was not limited to Jesus himself. It was always Jesus' plan to expand the Kingdom and the deliverance, healing, and salvation that went with it. Three important scriptures show how that was to take place.

LUKE 9

In Luke 9 Jesus commissioned the Twelve to minister in his name. Incredibly, he gave them power and authority to drive out all demons and cure disease, and he sent them to preach the kingdom of God and heal the sick. The same power and authority that Jesus had been exercising, he gave to the Twelve. It became their mission to expand the Kingdom just as Jesus had done. It is important to note that he gave them both power and the authority to use it. They were to do the same work that Jesus had been doing. Satan does have power on the earth, but not all power. Jesus came to take back authority over the world, to reclaim it for the kingdom of heaven.

LUKE 10

In Luke 10 we see another expansion of the Kingdom. This time Jesus commissions not twelve but seventy-two disciples to carry on the work of the Kingdom. He told them, "The harvest is plentiful, but the workers are few. Ask the Lord of the harvest, therefore, to send out workers into his harvest field. Go!" (Luke 10:2–3). A few verses later, we see the

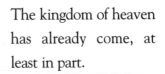

The kingdom of heaven has already come, at least in part.

result. The seventy-two returned with great joy saying, "Lord, even the demons submit to us in your name" (Luke 10:17). They were shocked, but they needn't have been. Jesus had given them authority to extend the Kingdom in his name. And with that authority came power. Jesus said in Matthew 12:28, "If I drive out demons by the Spirit of God, then the kingdom of God has come upon you." The fact that the seventy-two were able to drive out demons showed that the kingdom of heaven had come with power.

MATTHEW 16

In Matthew 16 we read Peter's classic confession of Christ. Jesus had gathered his disciples to ask them what was being said about him. "Who do people say that I am?" he asked. Various answers were given. Then Jesus put the question squarely to the disciples. In response, Peter made this declaration: "You are the Christ, the Son of the living God" (Matt. 16:16). Jesus replied, "Blessed are you, Simon son of Jonah, for this was not revealed to you by man, but by my Father in heaven. And I tell you that you are Peter, and on this rock I will build my church, and the gates of Hades will not overcome it. I will give you the keys of the kingdom of heaven; whatever you bind on earth will be bound in heaven, and whatever you loose on earth will be loosed in heaven" (Matt. 16:17–19).

With that incredible statement, Jesus transferred the same Kingdom power and authority that he had first given to the Twelve, then to the seventy-two, to the church—all believers. In other words, we are to go out and do exactly what Jesus had done: establish his Kingdom on earth, just as it is in heaven. We have been given that power and the authority to use it.

ON EARTH AS IT IS IN HEAVEN

Imagine a time when the kingdom of heaven has been fully established. Imagine a world without injustice, without pain, without suffering or tears or sickness. Imagine a new world in which everything and everyone is made whole. That is the heaven that we all long for. But that Kingdom is here now—at least in part. Jesus inaugurated that Kingdom with his ministry, and he passed on to us the power and authority to extend it. With the Kingdom comes deliverance, salvation, and healing. Jesus, who holds the keys to the Kingdom, has given those keys to us. And we are to exercise authority in his name.

Is there healing in heaven? Complete, ultimate healing? Yes, there is. And that healing is to begin here, now, in the kingdom of heaven that Jesus established. The kingdom of heaven is coming, yet, at the same time, it is already here. And with that Kingdom there will be healing here and now. As Jesus taught us, let us pray that God's kingdom shall continue to come and that his will shall continue to be done here on earth, just as it is in heaven.

LET'S PRAY

Father—

I am longing for heaven. I picture the day when there will be no more tears, pain, or sorrow. I wish it were today. And I thank you for giving me a glimpse of what you will do—a preview of the life that is to come. Help me to be a faithful messenger of your good news. Enable me to tell others about Jesus and to pray for those who need your healing power. I want to be your servant.

In Jesus' name I ask this.

Amen.

For small group discussion questions on this chapter and additional resources on healing, visit www.wesleyan.org/gsh.

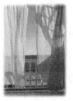

DOESN'T GOD USE SICKNESS TO TEACH PEOPLE?

God wants to teach us through his Word,
not through sickness.

Roberta's cancer had returned after a four-year absence. Within weeks it had spread throughout her body, requiring intense and painful treatments. She sat in her hospital room fighting nausea and trying to sleep. The door swung open to reveal Jeff Arnold, the pastor from Roberta's church.

"How are you feeling, Roberta?" Jeff pulled up a chair beside her bed and sat down.

"I don't know, Pastor. I guess I'm just sick of being sick."

She stared out the window. "I wish I didn't have to go through this."

"But remember what the Bible says, Roberta. All things work together for good in your life—even your disease."

Roberta said nothing.

"And you don't want to miss out on God's blessing. Doesn't James tell us to count it all joy when we face trials. That means you." The pastor's face brightened. "I can't wait to see what God is teaching you through this cancer!"

Roberta felt ill. "Does God really want me to be sick?" she wondered. "What have I done to deserve this? Is something wrong with my faith?"

She forced a smile. "I guess you're right," she said meekly. "I just hope I learn my lesson soon."

Many Christians believe that God uses sickness and other forms of pain in order to teach them. According to this way of thinking, every bad thing that happens in the world is directed by God, who has a particular reason for doing so. If an earthquake destroys thousands of homes, killing hundreds of people, God did it for some reason. And when people get cancer or diabetes or arthritis, God must have some agenda in mind for them. He is using their illness to teach them a lesson. That's another way of saying that God doesn't want everyone to be well; he wants some people to be sick.

GOD WANTS YOU WELL

There are two problems with this thinking. One is that it simply doesn't make sense. After all, if it were the case that illness is God's way of getting people's attention, we would have to conclude that what the world needs is more illness. If that's the way God operates, why wouldn't he make everybody sick until they finally wised up and did what he wanted?

The second problem with that line of thought is that it doesn't fit with Scripture. That fact is that we *do* learn in the midst of sickness. But the question is this: does God inflict illness on people in order to teach them, or does he teach them in other ways? Let's look at the Word.

SICKNESS IS FROM THE DEVIL

The book of Acts is our record of the early church. It was written by Luke, a medical doctor, a little more than thirty years after Jesus ascended into heaven. Acts 10:38 says, "[You know] how God anointed Jesus of Nazareth with the Holy Spirit and power, and how he went around doing good and healing all who were under the power of the devil, because God was with him." Who is responsible for inflicting sickness on people? According to the Bible, the devil is responsible for making people ill. There's no room in this text for the suggestion that making people ill is something God does.

> Disease and destruction are the work of the devil, and Jesus came to destroy the devil's work.

It is true that we learn a lot when we are sick. That is because we are in a humble condition and our minds are easily focused on things of ultimate importance. We live in a broken world, and we see that very clearly when we are suffering. But the Bible never suggests that God says, "Maybe if I give this child lupus he'll learn some things and honor me more." God simply doesn't do that. Sickness is from the devil, not from God.

JESUS HAS AN OPPOSITE AGENDA

If the devil uses illness to keep people in his power, what does Jesus do? What is his agenda in the world? John 10:10 spells that out clearly. Jesus said, "The thief comes only to steal and kill and destroy; I have come that they may have life, and have it to the full." Jesus drew the lines quite clearly. Satan wants to harm people and, ultimately, destroy them. Jesus wants to give them life. The devil wants people to be sick; Jesus wants them well.

The book of 1 John was written in about A.D. 95 by Jesus' good friend and disciple, John. If anyone knew Jesus well, it was John, often referred to as the beloved disciple. John wrote, "He who does what is sinful is of the devil, because the devil has been sinning from the beginning. The reason the Son of God appeared was to destroy the devil's work" (1 John 3:8). The ministry of Jesus was to destroy the work of the devil, so what did Jesus do? He preached the good news, healed people, and delivered them. The ministry of Jesus was centered on breaking the power of the Enemy over the human heart, mind, and body. Jesus came to heal people, not to make them ill.

JESUS CAME TO HEAL

Does Jesus want people to be sick? No, quite the opposite. The stated agenda for his ministry is to make people well. While it is also true that we learn a great deal when we suffer, the infliction of illness is *not* God's strategy for teaching us. God doesn't make people sick in order to get their attention or teach them a lesson. Sickness is the work of the Enemy. God wants you well.

THE RIGHT PICTURE OF GOD

When I was a child living in rural Kansas, one of the biggest events in life was when the fire truck went by. When I heard the siren and the roar of the engine, I knew something exciting was happening. It was such a big event in the small town near our farm that whenever the fire truck pulled out of the station, people would follow it. Back then we didn't know we weren't supposed to do that, so any fire became a gathering of the whole community. As a child, I saw a fire truck on a couple of occasions. Each time, it was parked in front of a burning house. Do you know what I concluded? I was convinced that firemen start fires in order to burn down houses. Why? Because the fire truck was always present when a house was on fire. It sounds silly now, but what else would a child think?

That mistaken logic is the same thinking that we apply to the issue of illness. When we see some trauma, illness, disaster, or even death, we also see the Holy Spirit at work. But the *presence* of the Holy Spirit does not mean he is the *cause*. We do learn when we are ill. The Holy Spirit helps us when we are traumatized. So we mistakenly conclude that God brought the trauma. We assume that it is God's job to inflict pain so that he will be able to offer comfort. Nothing could be further from the truth. And when we understand the nature of God, we will know that he is a merciful God who does not wish for his children to suffer any more than I, as an earthly father, want my children to suffer.

A GOD OF MERCY

Charles Capps once explained this truth using the following fictitious story. Suppose a man broke his leg and had to spend some time in the hospital, and when someone visited him, he said, "Praise God! He knew I needed a rest." What kind of God would break a man's leg in order to get him to take a day off? If God did half of the things he is accused of doing, he could be charged with child abuse! Would any of us tell our children that they need to go rest in their rooms, then break their legs in order to make them stay there? Certainly there must be a better way for God to teach us.

One day Jesus encountered a man who was possessed by demons (see Luke 8:26–39). This man was in such desperate condition that he wore no clothes and lived alone in the graveyard. People had tried to confine him with chains, but when the demons seized him he became violent, broke free, and ran. Now Jesus set this man free from the demons. He was so grateful for what Jesus had done that he wanted to accompany Jesus as one of his disciples.

Based on Scripture, how does God teach people, by inflicting sickness on them or by setting them free from disease? Here's another question: what is a more effective means of teaching people, torturing them or showing them mercy?

God intends to teach us not by inflicting pain but by relieving it. He teaches us by showing mercy. His plan is to heal us.

A GOD OF COMPASSION

People have come up with various explanations for the source of God's healing power. Some, basing their argument on Isaiah 53:4–5, contend that the Atonement (Christ's death on the cross) is our source of healing. The Bible says that Christ was "pierced for our transgressions" and "crushed for our iniquities," and that "by his wounds we are healed." Based on those statements, some believe that Jesus' death is the source of our healing. Yet if that were true, everyone who came to God for healing would receive it, just as all who come to God for salvation are freely forgiven.

> God is a loving father who gives good gifts to his children.

Others believe that God's healing accompanies his Kingdom. While I am not certain it is accurate to say that healing is in the Atonement, I believe it is inaccurate to say that healing is in the Kingdom. Based on the life and ministry of Jesus, they see wherever the reign of God is established, there will be healing. I agree with this viewpoint. Yet the Kingdom has not yet *fully* come. Jesus inaugurated the Kingdom, and it continues to expand. But it will not be fully established until Christ returns.

The ultimate source of our healing is neither in the Atonement nor in the Kingdom. It is in the compassionate nature of God. Jesus said,

"When he saw the crowds, he had compassion on them, because they were harassed and helpless, like sheep without a shepherd" (Matt. 9:36). Compassion pours from those words. It is the compassion of a Father, brokenhearted over the suffering of the world. It is the compassion of a Son who begs for more helpers to relieve the suffering he sees around him. Yes, we learn when we are ill. But we cannot conclude that our loving Heavenly Father *sends* disease in order to teach us.

A GOD OF GRACE

Many insurance policies excludes certain things called "acts of God." What are those? They are such things as tornadoes, hurricanes, and hailstorms. Is that really an accurate picture of God's "acts"? Is God someone who inflicts disaster upon us? Is calamity what God uses to teach us?

In fact, disasters of that kind are the work of the Enemy. How does God want to teach us? How does a good dad want his kids to learn? Would an earthly father rather have his children learn by being punished or by listening to their father's word? And that's the way God teaches us—through his Word. He has given us patient instruction in Scripture. He has given us the example and teaching of his Son, Jesus Christ. And he has given us the Counselor, the Holy Spirit, who guides and directs us. God's Word is his means of instructing his children.

Certainly, there are times when God instructs his children and they disobey him. And there are occasions when he instructs them again, and they disobey again. Finally, God may say, "All right, I'm going to have to let my children learn the hard way," and allow them to follow their own will. That always brings disaster. Do we learn in the midst of sickness, heartache and pain that we experience as a result of disobeying God? Of course we learn. But it is never God's will for us that we should suffer only to learn something. And none of us would say that we prefer to learn the hard way. God instructs us through his Word because he cares about us. He is a God of grace.

A GOD OF LOVE

I once heard Charles Capps give a powerful illustration of this truth. A couple whose child had been born with a severe deformity was interviewed on television. They said, "We don't know why God did this, but we were lucky to find a plastic surgeon who could correct it." We would feel compassion for this family and their child, but we would be saddened by their poor understanding of who God is. How much better it would have been if they said: "We don't understand how or why the Enemy has inflicted this suffering upon our child. But we praise God that he has given knowledge and skill to physicians and has given us the resources to provide for our child's care so that she can be made well."

Sickness is the work of Satan. It is the Enemy who has come to steal and kill and destroy. Healing is the work of God. It is Jesus who has come to give life and to give it abundantly. Your Heavenly Father loves you intensely. Never doubt his compassion, his mercy, and his love for you. We can thank God that we have learned when we are ill. Yet we can thank him even more that he is the God who heals.

LET'S PRAY

Father—

Thank you for your great love for me. Thank you for your compassion, mercy, and grace. I need to know that you love me, especially when I am in pain. Relieve my doubts, Father, and enable me to rest in my faith. I love you, and I trust you.

In Jesus' name I pray,

Amen.

For small group discussion questions on this chapter and additional resources on healing, visit www.wesleyan.org/gsh.

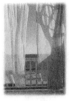

IF YOU HAVE THE GIFT, WHY NOT EMPTY THE HOSPITAL?

Not every person is ready to receive God's healing.

⬥⬥⬥

Don and Karl met for prayer every Tuesday morning. They resisted the term accountability partners, *but the close friends made a habit of challenging each other to be spiritually authentic. Lately Don had been seeking God's guidance about determining his spiritual gifts.*

"I've been praying a lot about it, Karl, and I sense that God wants me to pray for the sick."

"Really?" Karl sounded a little surprised.

"Yeah," Don continued, "in fact, I've been doing that pretty often lately. I actually healed someone."

Karl raised an eyebrow. "Oh?"

"Well, God healed her, actually. It was my niece. She had the flu, and I prayed for her. Her fever broke within minutes. She went to school the next day."

"The flu, huh?"

"I know it sounds hokey, but she was really sick." Don paused. "I think I may have the gift of healing."

"OK," Karl said. "Let's go."

"Go? Where?"

"To the hospital. You've got the gift of healing, right? Let's go clear the place out."

"Um . . . I'm not so sure about that," Don said weakly. "Let's have another cup of coffee."

If you have the gift of healing, then why wouldn't you make everyone well? That's a reasonable question. A compassionate person who was able to exercise the gift of healing would certainly want to do so whenever possible. If it really is a simple matter to pray for healing, why hasn't someone gone to the hospital and emptied the place? Many hospitals are filled, and some have waiting lists. Some people assume that because some sick people are not healed, divine healing must not be real.

There are reasons, however, why some people are not healed. A number of those reasons will be treated in the third section of this book. For now, let's look specifically at divine healing applied in the setting of a hospital. Why don't we simply visit a hospital, pray for healing, and empty every bed? To answer that question, let's examine an occasion on which Jesus visited something very much like a hospital. The story is recorded in John 5:1–8.

Some time later, Jesus went up to Jerusalem for a feast of the Jews. Now there is in Jerusalem near the Sheep Gate a pool, which in Aramaic is called Bethesda and which is surrounded by five covered colonnades. Here a great number of disabled people used to lie—the blind, the lame, the paralyzed. One who was there had been an invalid for thirty-eight years. When Jesus saw him lying there and learned that he had been in this condition for a long time, he asked him, "Do you want to get well?"

"Sir," the invalid replied, "I have no one to help me into the pool when the water is stirred. While I am trying to get in, someone else goes down ahead of me."

Then Jesus said to him, "Get up! Pick up your mat and walk." At once the man was cured; he picked up his mat and walked.

READY TO RECEIVE

The pool at Bethesda was the ancient equivalent of a hospital or nursing home. People believed that an angel would occasionally stir the water in that pool, then the first person to enter it would be healed. Many sick people congregated near the pool, hoping to get their chance at healing. When Jesus arrived he encountered a man who had been sick for thirty-eight years. Notice the question that Jesus asked the man: "Do you want to get well?"

This poor man totally missed the point of Jesus' question. He replied, "There's no one to take me to the pool."

But Jesus didn't ask, "Do you have anybody to take you to the pool?" He didn't even ask, "Why are you still sick?" If Jesus had asked either of those questions, then saying "There's no one to help me into the pool" would have been a good answer.

But Jesus asked, "Do you want to get well?" To that question, the obvious answer would be, "Yes! I want to be well." But the man didn't say that. He ignored Jesus' question and talked instead about the obstacles to his healing.

There are several reasons why people may not be ready to receive the gift of healing.

Jesus was asking a more fundamental question than "Why are you ill?" or "Do you need help?" He was getting into the heart of the diseased person. His question got to the issue of the will. Did the man really want to be well? Doesn't everyone? One would suppose that they do, but in fact, there are reasons why some people are unwilling or unready to receive the gift of divine healing.

A LOSS OF HOPE

Jesus' question to the man at the pool is perhaps confrontational. Is may seem impolite to question whether or not sick people really want healing, but Jesus asked. He knew that when people are sick for a long time, they can come to accept their circumstances, assuming that things will never change. It is possible that they quit even looking for a solution to their problem. They accept a lifestyle of illness. They lose hope.

You may have seen examples of that attitude. I saw it once in a lady named Linda. She was a former staff member for a nationwide parachurch organization and was a very fine Christian lady. Yet as a child, her mother had involved her and her sister in seances in their home. The spirit of destruction entered Linda at a young age. After she began working for the parachurch ministry, it began to reoccur, causing severe emotional and physical problems. Linda could clearly trace these problems to the time when she was about eight years old and the Enemy entered her life.

On one occasion I said, "Linda, this problem isn't too big for God. Let us pray for you." By doing that, I was asking something like "Do you want to be well?"

Linda said, "Jim, every time I try to get release from this, I suffer so much. It's hardly worth trying anymore. I've learned to cope with this, and I just live with it."

I said, "Linda, please don't give up. Please, let us pray for you." She said, "No."

That response is more common that you might think. There are many people who have simply given up on the idea of divine healing because they have experienced pain for so long and have had many disappointments. They don't want to be prayed for anymore. It is understandable when that happens, but it is also tragic. Many people who are in a hospital or are living in a nursing home have simply accepted their condition. They love God and believe in him. Yet they have come to believe that they will never be healed. That thought pattern is one reason why it is not possible to simply empty the hospitals with prayer for healing.

A SOURCE OF POWER

A second reason why we do not heal every hospitalized person has to do with the motivation of some sick people. After I had preached a sermon on divine healing, someone handed me a note. In that sermon I had mentioned some reasons why people aren't healed, and a person wrote a note to suggest one more. The note read: "One block to healing is the personal gratification of the sick person. If healed, that person will have no way to get personal attention."

That probably applies to very few people, but it might apply to some. There are some sick people who actually embrace their condition because of the status it affords them with friends or relatives. And that is one reason why it is unrealistic to expect that a person with the gift of healing could instantly heal every person he or she encountered. The sick person must want to be made well.

A DIFFICULT ENVIRONMENT

Another reason we cannot miraculously empty the hospital is that it is one of the most intimidating environments in which to pray for the sick. That statement may be surprising. You might think that a place filled with sick people would be ideal ground to exercise the gift of healing, yet it is not.

For one thing, the hospital is not our turf as nonprofessionals in the medical field. It is the turf of doctors, nurses, and other health care professionals. When we go to a hospital to pray for the sick, we are under their authority and are understandably asked to wait, step aside, or leave the room while the medical people perform their work.

Yet the hospital is not, ultimately, the territory even of medical professionals; in one sense it is the territory of the Enemy. It was under John Wimber's teaching that I first began to understand this. A hospital is a place of compassionate work. In fact, many hospitals carry the names of Christian saints because they were established by Christian people who were motivated by Jesus' call to compassion. There are many doctors and nurses who treat patients with incredible love and concern. Yet what is the source of sickness? It is not God but the Enemy who makes people ill (see chapter 7). So there is a sense in which the collection of sick and diseased people in a hospital are a sort of trophy for the Enemy. To be sure, I'm not speaking about the hearts of the people working or receiving treatment there. But hospitals clearly display the trauma caused by the Enemy on the human body. For that reason, it can be a very challenging place to pray for the sick. In spite of that, we do go to hospitals and pray for healing there. We must not allow ourselves to be intimidated by the fact that hospitals are not our home territory. We go there to pray, and we do see healing. Yet we recognize that it can be a challenging environment in which to pray.

A Connection with the Father

A final reason we do not simply empty the hospitals with our prayer for healing is that we are to join God in his ministry of healing, not direct it. In my opinion—and this may surprise you—God has not directed us to pray for healing at all times and in all places. Rather, we are to participate in Jesus' ministry of healing, wherever and whenever that is taking place.

> Our job is not to heal everyone. It is to see what the Father is doing and join him in it.

When we pray for healing, we don't simply run from one sick person to another, laying hands on people as fast as we can. We make an effort to see what the Father is doing. That may mean that there are occasions when we do not offer prayer for a sick person. Does that mean it is not God's will for everybody to be healed? I believe it is his desire for every person to be well, but we accomplish that by joining God in his timing. That's why we don't simply walk the corridors at a hospital, laying hands on people whether they are interested in healing prayer or not. We see where the Father is working and join him.

Hope for Healing

Do you want to be well? The question may seem rhetorical, but Jesus asked it of at least one sick person. Are there people who do not want to be well? It might be more accurate to say that some are not ready to receive the gift of God's healing power. And God will not dispense his grace to those who are not ready—for whatever reason—to accept it.

Yet we can pray this prayer for every person who is sick, and for ourselves. We can pray that God would make them ready to receive his grace, whether it be in the form of salvation from sin, deliverance from bondage, or healing from disease. We can ask that he would make their hearts ready to receive the gift that he is so willing to give.

LET'S PRAY

Father—

I want to be an instrument of healing in the lives of others. I want to pray so that others may be well. Help me to see where my prayers may be most effective. Give me a sense of your purpose in every situation, so that I may see your will and pray in harmony with it. Give me discernment, Lord.

In Jesus' name I pray,

Amen.

———— ❀ ————

For small group discussion questions on this chapter and additional resources on healing, visit www.wesleyan.org/gsh.

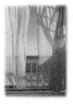

NINE

IF HEALING WERE REAL, WOULDN'T IT BE INSTANTANEOUS?

While instantaneous healing does occur,
most healing comes gradually.

Testimony time at Seth's church was as predictable as the result of a Cubs game. Pastor Baker tried valiantly to elicit some report of a fresh conversion, miracle, or other work of the Spirit, but most members used the occasion to make announcements or trot out the same old requests for prayer.

Seth winced as Martha Carter rose to her feet. Everyone knew all about her gall stones, arthritis, and chronic urinary tract infections.

"I'd like to thank the Lord for his healing power,"
Martha began. "He touched me this week."

Seth rolled his eyes. "It's about time," he muttered under
his breath.

"I've been praying about my arthritis for over a year,"
Martha continued.

"And you've been on medication, had surgery, and been
through physical therapy," Seth thought impatiently. "We
know all that."

"And this week, I was able to walk without using my
cane," Martha said triumphantly. "I praise God for what
he's done in me." Then she sat down.

"What God's done?" Seth wondered. Seems like she
should be thanking her doctor. I can't see where God did any-
thing."

M ost of the healings recorded in the Bible occurred immediately.
Scripture is filled with reports of lepers being healed in an instant,
blind people having their sight restored all at once, and even dead people being raised to life. Other types of miracles seem to have happened
suddenly also. When Moses led the
Hebrew people out of slavery, he
stretched out his rod over the Red Sea,
and the waters parted. One moment, the
people faced a vast body of water. The
next moment, they were walking across
that space on dry ground. So it seems logical to conclude that divine
healing is always an instantaneous transaction. That's the way miracles
happen, isn't it?

> We long for instant
> results, yet healing often
> takes time.

Healing as a Process

Remember, however, that when God sent Moses to deliver the Hebrew people, it was after four hundred years of bondage. God's deliverance was the culmination of a process that began when Joseph was sold into slavery, then promoted to the second-highest position in all of Egypt. The deliverance seemed to come all at once, but it was actually centuries in the making.

And what about the miracles themselves? Did they always happen instantly? Did any miracles happen gradually? There are at least three examples in Scripture of people who were healed or delivered through a process that took place over time. Let's look at each of them.

A Two-Stage Healing

Perhaps the clearest example of this kind of miracle occurred in a place called Bethsaida, where Jesus healed a blind man in two distinct stages. Mark 8:22–25 provides this account:

> They came to Bethsaida, and some people brought a blind man and begged Jesus to touch him. He took the blind man by the hand and led him outside the village. When he had spit on the man's eyes and put his hands on him, Jesus asked, "Do you see anything?"
>
> He looked up and said, "I see people; they look like trees walking around."
>
> Once more Jesus put his hands on the man's eyes. Then his eyes were opened, his sight was restored, and he saw everything clearly.

This is the best example in Scripture of healing as a process. Although the Bible doesn't explain why he did so, Jesus healed the man in two stages. It is true that the stages came close together, and the whole process probably took no more than a minute or two; but the healing came gradually, not in one instant.

GRADUAL HEALING

Another Scripture passage gives us a snapshot of healing that is not instantaneous. This event occurred over both time and distance, as Jesus healed a boy gradually who was lying ill in another place. The event is recorded John 4:46–53. The New American Standard Bible renders it this way:

> Therefore He came again to Cana of Galilee where He had made the water wine And there was a royal official whose son was sick at Capernaum.
>
> When he heard that Jesus had come out of Judea into Galilee, he went to Him and was imploring Him to come down and heal his son; for he was at the point of death.
>
> So Jesus said to him, "Unless you people see signs and wonders, you simply will not believe."
>
> The royal official said to Him, "Sir, come down before my child dies."
>
> Jesus said to him, "Go; your son lives." The man believed the word that Jesus spoke to him and started off.
>
> As he was now going down, his slaves met him, saying that his son was living.
>
> So he inquired of them the hour when he began to get better. Then they said to him, "Yesterday at the seventh hour the fever left him."
>
> So the father knew that it was at that hour in which Jesus said to him, "Your son lives"; and he himself believed and his whole household.

Notice the phrase, "when he began to get better." That is one of the few passages of Scripture that might suggest that a divine healing came gradually. Jesus healed the boy, without question. But it seems that the child may not have become well immediately. The healing likely took place over a short period of time. We don't know how long the time was, but the language of the text seems to indicate that the healing was not instantaneous; it may have come over time.

DELAYED DELIVERANCE

There is another example in Scripture of a miracle that did not take place all at once. This one is not an account of healing but of deliverance. In a place called the Gerasenes, Jesus delivered a man from demon possession; but the deliverance came after a slight delay. Mark 5:1–13 reports:

They went across the lake to the region of the Gerasenes. When Jesus got out of the boat, a man with an evil spirit came from the tombs to meet him. This man lived in the tombs, and no one could bind him any more, not even with a chain. For he had often been chained hand and foot, but he tore the chains apart and broke the irons on his feet. No one was strong enough to subdue him. Night and day among the tombs and in the hills he would cry out and cut himself with stones.

When he saw Jesus from a distance, he ran and fell on his knees in front of him. He shouted at the top of his voice, "What do you want with me, Jesus, Son of the Most High God? Swear to God that you won't torture me!" For Jesus had said to him, "Come out of this man, you evil spirit!"

Then Jesus asked him, "What is your name?"

"My name is Legion," he replied, "for we are many." And he begged Jesus again and again not to send them out of the area.

A large herd of pigs was feeding on the nearby hillside. The demons begged Jesus, "Send us among the pigs; allow us to go into them." He gave them permission, and the evil spirits came out and went into the pigs. The herd, about two thousand in number, rushed down the steep bank into the lake and were drowned.

This story is interesting for several reasons. It was just prior to this event that Jesus stilled a storm on the Sea of Galilee. Jesus was on his way to the Gerasenes by boat when a fierce storm arose. The Enemy was trying to sink the boat by tampering with the weather patterns, but Jesus put a stop to that by rebuking the wind and waves. How do we know it was the Enemy? Is it possible that the storm was sent by God? No, it is not possible because Jesus rebuked the storm. Since Jesus is always in agreement with the Father, he would not stop something the Father had started. Jesus came to undo the works of the devil.

Then, shortly after that encounter with evil, Jesus came upon this poor man, who is probably the most demonized person in Scripture. The man was in such a pathetic condition that he lived out among the tombs, naked, crying out and cutting himself with stones.

Notice the interchange between this demon-possessed man and Jesus. It's a spiritual tug-of-war as Jesus commands the demons to come out but they initially refuse. Fearing Jesus' power, the demons actually bargain with him! Finally, Jesus allows the demons to enter a herd of pigs, which immediately rushes into the lake and is drowned. Ironically, that is the same body of water, in which the Enemy had just tried to drown Jesus!

The important point for us to note is that there is a delay between the time that Jesus commands the demons to leave the man and the moment when the fellow is actually delivered. We're used to the idea that miracles happen instantly. In this case there appears to have been a momentary delay.

Unity with the Father

Francis McNutt, a Catholic priest who has been involved with healing for many years, estimates that fewer than 20 percent of the cases of divine healing he has witnessed were instantaneous. About 50 percent were gradual, and at least one quarter of the people he has prayed for did not get better at all. Those estimates are probably a good reflection of the experience of divine healing in our day. Is it frustrating that more people are not healed and that they are not healed instantly? Could we wish that more people were healed immediately, as is recorded so often in the Bible? Certainly. Yet it seems that in our day, God most often chooses to heal people gradually or after some delay—sometimes a very long delay. I myself was healed of a respiratory condition that troubled me for thirteen long years. Approximately one year before publishing this book, my long-desired healing came. I concede that the "delays" in Scripture may have been but a few moments, and I cannot explain the lengthy delays in many instances of contemporary healing. Yet those delays will not deter me from continuing to pray for healing.

> For reasons that I can't fully explain, God most often chooses to heal gradually.

Are there possible explanations as to why Jesus nearly always healed people instantly while most healing today takes place gradually? Part of the reason is the purity of heart of Jesus. He had oneness with the Father and was able to see clearly what the Father was doing. Also, the healing ministry of Jesus and his disciples was empowered by much prayer and fasting. Could it be that we do not see more instantaneous healing because we are less united with the Father and less empowered through prayer and fasting?

I'm tremendously encouraged by the amount of healing that I see taking place today. Yet almost all of it is happening gradually. Instantaneous healing does occur, but, for whatever reason, God chooses now to heal most people through a process, over time. For those who are suffering, gradual healing is certainly better than none at all. If this is the way God chooses to work, we should accept it gratefully.

Let us also strengthen our unity with the Father. Let's seek a pure heart, a greater connection to the heart of God, and dedicate ourselves to prayer and fasting for divine healing. I believe we will see God work in a mighty way.

LET'S PRAY

Father—

I admit that I am impatient. I long to see your power released in mighty ways—right now. I struggle to be persistent and faithful in praying for healing when there seems to be no result. Lord, give me the fruit of patience. Help me to trust you without wavering. And, Father, I ask you to bless me and those around me with life and health.

In Jesus' name,

Amen.

For small group discussion questions on this chapter and additional resources on healing, visit www.wesleyan.org/gsh.

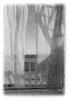

WHAT ABOUT PEOPLE WHO AREN'T HEALED?

*Sometimes we simply don't know
why a person isn't healed.*

Pastor Jared never went to the post office without running into a parishioner or two. Usually they wanted to stop and chat, which meant it always took a little longer to run errands. But Jared considered it ministry time. Often, he wound up praying for people at the hardware store or in the park.

He met Louise Blanchard as he stepped away from his post office box.

"I've been praying for your mom, Louise," he said gently. The older woman had been battling cancer for nearly two years.

Louise said nothing. Tears welled in her eyes.

Jared laid a hand on her shoulder. "It's hard, isn't it?" he offered.

A pause.

"I hope this won't make you uncomfortable, Louise, but I'd like to pray for your mom right now. Would that be all right?"

Louise struggled to get the words out, barely able to contain her emotions.

"No, pastor," she stammered. "There's no need for that now . . . Mom's gone."

"I'm sorry," Jared said.

"It's OK, pastor," Louise said, brushing tears from her cheek. "I guess God wanted her more than we do—that's why he took her away."

What about the people who aren't healed? If God still heals, then why are some people *not* healed? Usually when we ask that question, we're thinking of someone in particular—a father, a wife, or a child. This question is a very personal one because all of us experience loss. The people we love may become ill and die. Why doesn't God heal them?

It would be impossible to consider every circumstance where a loved one did not receive healing. But the Bible does give a few clear and well-known examples of people who coped with illness and were not healed or were not healed immediately. Perhaps these cases have come to mind as you've considered your own illness or that of a loved one. What about Job? What about Paul? What about Timothy? They were certainly godly people. If anyone deserves healing, they did. Yet they were not healed. Why not?

Let's consider these cases and a few others. As we do, we'll uncover some common misconceptions about divine healing, and we'll learn that in spite of the fact that some people aren't healed, God is still a healer and we can continue to rely on his grace. We'll begin with the story of Job because that particular book of the Bible voices the question that so often comes to our minds when we wonder why people aren't healed: Why do bad things happen to good people?

JOB

The book of Job isn't just a story. He was an actual person who lived in the land of Uz. Job was a blameless man. Various translations of the Bible use different words to describe Job, but all translators emphasize the fact that Job was a good man. That doesn't mean he was faultless or had never sinned. It simply means that so far as his heart was concerned, he was right with God. He was pure in spirit.

Yet Job was besieged by problems. As you may know, the Enemy asked for and received God's permission to afflict Job with a series of tragedies. First, Job's possessions were taken from him, then his children. All of them fell victim to calamity in a single day. Later, Job himself was afflicted with painful sores all over his body. In spite of the fact that Job was blameless before God, he suffered many things including illness.

Early in the book of Job, we find a statement that is often recited by those who suffer. However, this well-known verse offers a poor understanding of the Father. Job loved God, but did not fully understand him—as the rest of the book makes abundantly clear. Immediately after receiving the bad news about the loss of his family, Job says, "Naked I came from my mother's womb, and naked I will depart. The LORD gave and the LORD has taken away; may the name of the LORD be praised" (Job 1:21). That thought is often shortened when used during a funeral and is rendered something like this: "The Lord gives, and the Lord takes away."

Is that true?

THE LORD TAKES?

The Bible is the inspired Word of God. However, in some passages it includes statements made by people who did not know the truth and which do not represent God's nature. In that sense, we can say that not every statement recorded in the Bible is true. Remember that the Bible includes the actions, thoughts, and statements of many ungodly people, including the Enemy. Not every person who speaks in the Bible is speaking for God. Even some of the devout people whose words are recorded in Scripture said things in error (as we'll see of Job a bit later). Some words and thoughts are recorded to show us what is *not* in keeping with the mind of God. Job's friends, for example, make outlandish claims that certainly are not true. At the end of the book, God steps in to correct them. Their words stand in contrast to the mind of God, not in agreement with it. So just because Job makes this statement does not mean that God intends for us to own it as truth.

> To consult a doctor or take medicine is *not* a denial of faith.

At first glance, the idea that "God gives and God takes away" seems right. It does seem to fit well at a funeral because there we are trying to cope with the loss of a loved one. Often, we are asking the question voiced in this chapter: Why aren't some people healed? It seems comforting to believe that they weren't healed because God took them. But think about that for a moment. Does that fit with what we know about God? It is God who blesses and gives life. Is it God who routinely takes life away from good people? Can you imagine God looking over a group of his beloved children and saying, "Hmm. I think I'll snatch life away from this one"?

Who is the one who introduced sickness and death into the human race? It was not God. It is the thief who comes to steal and kill and destroy; God is the giver of life (see John 10:10). Job is simply mistaken when he assigns responsibility for killing innocent people to God. That is the work of the Enemy.

I lost a sister to illness and a brother to a plane crash many years ago. I reviewed some of the things that were sent to my parents upon the deaths of their children. Many of them were very tender thoughts and were expressed with the best motives, but they were simply wrong. After the death of my sister Janie, someone sent a card that read, "She was a beautiful rose, and God reached down from heaven and picked it."

I do not, however, believe that statement. We live in a world that is broken and filled with heartache, and heartache is from the Enemy. God does not inflict unspeakable grief upon two wonderful parents by striking their innocent child dead. Death came through the work of Satan. It is the work of the Enemy. In fact, before Satan's sin, there was no sickness or death. God created a world that was originally free from these things. The Lord is the giver of good gifts.

THE SELF-FULFILLING POWER OF FEAR

In Job 3:25–26, Job says, "What I feared has come upon me; what I dreaded has happened to me. I have no peace, no quietness; I have no rest, but only turmoil." Job was blameless, but he wasn't faultless. He was an upstanding man who undoubtedly lived a good life. But he lived a long time ago, long before the time of Christ. In fact, the book of Job is believed to be the oldest book in the Bible. All of that means that Job did not have access to the revelation that has been given since that time. He did not have the Old Testament to read, let alone the words of Christ. So his understanding of truth as you and I know it was primitive. And when Job says, "What I feared has come upon me," he is admitting the fact that he has given in to a spirit of fear. Over and over again, the Bible says things like "Do not be afraid." Fear is the opposite of faith. Fear cripples us and allows the Enemy a foothold in our lives. Faith releases the Spirit of God to work on our behalf. As some of us occasionally do, Job allowed himself to be overtaken by fear.

Don't allow fear to come upon you. Don't live with the mindset that something dreadful is going to befall you. When you do, you open your life for the Enemy to attack through your fear. Instead, choose not to fear because you are filled with the confidence that comes through faith.

GOD SLAYS HIM?

Another often-quoted statement by Job is found in Job 13:15. Job says, "Though he slay me, yet will I hope in him." That verse is usually quoted as an affirmation of faith in the face of adversity. It is a favorite of many godly people, so I realize that my comments about it may be unpopular. Yet the premise of Job's statement is incorrect. I am referring to the words "though he slay me." Remember that it is not God who slays the innocent. Certainly God can snuff out the lives of the wicked, and some scriptures support that. But God is the giver of life, and he gives it abundantly to all who believe. God loves you. More than that, he *likes* you and desires your company. He does not come to slay us but to heal us. It is the Enemy who inflicts harm, heartache, and death. So Job's statement would have been much more accurate if he had said something like this, "In spite of the fact that the Enemy has destroyed my family and inflicted great pain upon me, I will continue to trust God and believe that he will deliver me, because I know he loves me."

At the end of the story, God steps in to challenge Job, and Job admits that he did not know what he had been talking about (Job 42:3). It is the Enemy who kills; God is the giver of life.

JOB REALIZES HIS ERROR

Remember that we're discussing the question "What about those who aren't healed?" Job's story is often used to support the argument that God actually wants some people to be ill. If God inflicted illness upon Job, they reason, then God must want some people to be sick. That's the basic line of thought pursued by three of Job's "comforters," the friends who came to counsel him about his problems. Their counsel boils down to this advice: Obviously you've done something terribly wrong, or else God wouldn't be punishing you by inflicting illness upon you. Do the right thing and confess your sins, then God will heal you.

Job's response to his friends emphasizes three points. Job says, in effect, (1) God doesn't hear my cries for help, (2) I haven't done anything wrong, but God is persecuting me anyway, and (3) It's not fair that God lets the wicked prosper. Job was suffering a great deal, and all of us have probably felt as he did when he suffered. You may feel that way now. God just doesn't seem fair.

For thirty-seven chapters of the book of Job, God remains silent while Job and his friends argue. Finally, God speaks. His answer can be summarized in two points. God says, basically, (1) I'm in control of the whole world, and (2) You're not. Ironically, God does not address the primary question that Job and his friends have been asking, "Why did this happen?" Instead, God asserts that he alone is sovereign and that his judgments are beyond question.

At that point Job recognizes his error. He says, "I am unworthy — how can I reply to you? I put my hand over my mouth. I spoke once, but I have no answer — twice, but I will say no more" (Job 40:4–5).

Job was humble enough that he was willing to admit that he was wrong in assigning God blame for the suffering in the world. Are we?

JOB BEGINS TO UNDERSTAND

Job goes on to say, "I know that you can do all things; no plan of yours can be thwarted. You asked, 'Who is this that obscures my counsel without knowledge?' Surely I spoke of things I did not understand, things too wonderful for me to know. You said, 'Listen now, and I will speak; I will question you, and you shall answer me.' My ears had heard of you but now my eyes have seen you. Therefore I despise myself and repent in dust and ashes" (Job 42:2–6). Incredibly, God then restored to Job everything that he had lost— possessions, servants, a new family, everything. In fact, by the end of his life, Job had twice the wealth that he had had at the beginning of the story. It was as if God said, "Now that you realize that I'm not out to get you, let me show you just how loving and generous I am."

WE SEE GOD'S MERCY

Many people use the book of Job to make the case that God wants some people to be sick. But Scripture itself tells us that that is not the case. One of the most basic principles for interpreting the Bible is that we allow the Bible to interpret itself. So our under-standing of the book of Job is clarified by the book of James, which comments on Job. James was the brother of Jesus and became the leader of the church in Jerusalem. James wrote, "As you know, we consider blessed those who have persevered. You have heard of Job's perseverance and have seen what the Lord finally brought about. The Lord is full of compassion and mercy" (James 5:11). James sees in the story of Job a portrait of God's compassion and mercy. God does not desire that his children should suffer. Instead, he enables them to persevere through the onslaught of attacks by the Enemy. Far from portraying God as the one who inflicts pain upon his children, the book of Job shows us clearly that God is the giver of good gifts.

Did God make his presence known early in Job's experience? No, he did not. In Job's circumstances, probably all of us would feel as Job did and would wonder where God was. But God does come, always, and when he comes, he makes his compassion known. Job teaches us that God is a God of mercy.

PAUL

Let's consider another biblical example, the Apostle Paul. Paul was the first great missionary of the Christian faith and a significant leader in the early church. His writing accounts for most of the books in the New Testament. Yet he dealt with a significant problem. In 2 Corinthians 12, Paul mentions that he suffered from a "thorn in the flesh." Paul wrote—

> To keep me from becoming conceited because of these surpassingly great revelations, there was given me a thorn in my flesh, a messenger of Satan, to torment me. Three times I pleaded with the Lord to take it away from me. But he said to me, 'My grace is sufficient for you, for my power is made perfect in weakness.' Therefore I will boast all the more gladly about my weaknesses, so that Christ's power may rest on me. That is why, for Christ's sake, I delight in weaknesses, in insults, in hardships, in persecutions, in difficulties. For when I am weak, then I am strong (2 Cor. 12:7–10).

Everyone agrees that the term *thorn in the flesh* is used as a metaphor, but people disagree on what the metaphor represents. For years some have argued that the thorn in the flesh was some chronic illness that Paul suffered. However, there is no evidence anywhere in Scripture that indicates that. Others think the "thorn" was Paul's poor eyesight. Perhaps the most unusual theory is that the term refers to Paul's mother-in-law! There are many interpretations of this term, but Scripture offers no hint that it was an illness.

THE 'THORN' IS NOT ILLNESS

Remember that Paul was Jewish. He understood and certainly used figures of speech that were drawn from Jewish culture. Every culture has idiomatic phrases. For example, when we say that the sun comes up in the morning, we are not saying that the earth is flat. We know the sun doesn't literally rise but that the earth revolves. To say that the sun rises is to use a figure of speech. Paul did the same in referring to the thorn in his flesh.

But what was he referring to? In the Old Testament, a similar phrase occurs three times. It is found in Numbers 33:55, Joshua 23:13, and Judges 2:3. In each case, the term *thorn* refers to ungodly people who are trying to stop the work of God, people who are wicked in their intentions. Now in 2 Corinthians 12, Paul uses this same term, *thorn*, and adds this description—"a messenger of Satan." Paul is borrowing a figure of speech from his Jewish culture—that of a thorn stuck into the body—by which he means to indicate some wicked person who is opposing the work of God. To make it more emphatic, he adds that this "thorn" is a messenger of Satan. So this passage does *not* indicate that Paul suffered from a physical illness but that he faced opposition from ungodly people. And we know that is true from Paul's other writings. He spoke often of the people who opposed the grace-filled message of the gospel, even calling them "dogs" at one point (Phil. 3:2).

Because many people interpret the term *thorn* to mean *illness,* it is commonly believed that God's word to Paul ("My grace is sufficient for you") really means something like, "Keep a stiff upper lip and keep fighting this illness." But if this thorn is not really an illness after all, then this advice to Paul must mean something different. What does it mean, in the context of opposition to the gospel, for God to say "My grace is sufficient"? What is grace? It is God's willingness to release his power on our behalf. So what God is really saying to Paul should be interpreted more like this: "Paul, if anyone knows about my power being released on your behalf, you do. *You* put on that power, and *you* put a stop to what the Enemy is doing."

PAUL CLAIMS GOD'S GRACE

Paul responded to God's admonition using the language of an ancient ceremony known as "cutting the covenant." When a king and a slave made a covenant, they shared their resources. Everything the wealthy king had was placed at the disposal of the poor slave. Paul, embracing covenantal language, said, in effect, "I am going to rejoice in how weak I am, because I know that I am partnered with God. So even though I am weak, I take on *his* strength!" Paul knew that with God, nothing is impossible. His words in 2 Corinthians 12 do not indicate that he had chosen to passively accept defeat in this area of his life. Instead, he claimed victory through the power of God.

We can do that too. Remember that illness is the work of the Enemy, so it is an opportunity for God to display his grace. Although Paul was not sick in this case, he showed us that we can claim God's strength when fighting against the Enemy. When we pray for healing, we do exactly that. It is interesting that nowhere in the New Testament does it say that we should contact God to get Satan to leave us alone. On the contrary, the New Testament teaches that *we* are to get rid of Satan when he harasses us by claiming God's authority.

TIMOTHY

Let's look at another biblical example, Timothy. This young associate of Paul was ill. We know that he had some stomach problems because Paul wrote to him saying, "Stop drinking only water, and use a little wine because of your stomach and your frequent illnesses" (1 Tim. 5:23). Some translations read "stomach ailments" in this passage. So timothy was instructed to use wine as medicine.

Timothy was a pastor. Our images of the early church often include the element of persecution. Indeed, persecution did come upon believers in those early days, so we often picture the fledgling church as a scattering of people hidden away in catacombs. But Timothy was a pastor during the boom years of the early church. In the city of Thessalonica alone there were perhaps as many as twenty thousand Christians. In Ephesus there may have been about fifty thousand believers. And in those days before the church was split up into many denominations, all believers in a city were part of a single congregation. And Timothy pastored at both Thessalonica and Ephesus before he was thirty years of age.

There is another pastor mentioned in Paul's letters: Titus. Timothy and Titus were as different as night and day. Titus was a bold, aggressive leader. He could tackle any problem, and nothing intimidated him. Timothy, on the other hand, had a more timid temperament. Titus and Paul constantly nudged Timothy forward. That came hard for Timothy, so he understandably had some stomach problems caused by stress. And believe me, if you are pastoring a church of some twenty thousand or more people, you're going to experience stress!

In those days, wine was commonly used as medicine, so Paul urged the young man to take some wine for his stomach. Telling Timothy to make use of an available treatment for his condition was good advice. It was not, however, an indication that God somehow *wanted* Timothy to he ill. Paul simply realized that dealing with life's problems can take a toll on the body. Paul was saying, in effect, "Take your medicine, Timothy."

What is the Scripture's view of medical treatment? If you go to a doctor or take medication, does that indicate a lack of faith? By taking an aspirin, are you admitting that God cannot heal you? Of course not!

Let's take a look at the story of Asa, king of Judah. In 2 Chronicles 16:12, we see that Asa was sick. He had a disease in his feet, and he consulted physicians rather than trusting God. Some have used that text to say that if you trust God, you will not consult a physician. But a closer look at the story reveals two things. First, the physicians Asa consulted were involved in witchcraft. Consulting someone who practices the occult is quite different from going to the doctor. Second, the problem was not that Asa consulted physicians but that he put his trust in them. While we may accept the medical advice of doctors, we do not put our ultimate faith in them. In fact, when I go to the doctor, I usually pray something like this: "Lord, I pray you'll show my physician things he may not even have learned in medical school. Help him to help me." I also pray that my physician will have a compassionate heart, as God does, and that he or she will gain supernatural insight in interpreting any tests I might undergo. I pray that way because I know that it is God who accomplishes my healing—sometimes using a doctor to do it.

> There is no need to defend God in cases where people have not been divinely healed. God doesn't need a lawyer.

There is nothing wrong with a Christian using medicine or consulting a doctor. Doing so is not a denial of faith. The fact that Paul told Timothy to take some wine for his stomach in no way indicates that God somehow wanted Timothy to be ill or had no intention of healing him. It was simply good advice from the seasoned apostle to his young friend. We have one evidence of Jesus using some type of "medicine." In the ancient world, saliva was sometimes seen as having healing properties. So it is significant that Jesus on occasion used saliva when performing a healing (see John 9:6). Here is the key point: there is no contest between believing in God's healing power and making us of medical science God wants us well, and sometimes medicine is what brings about our healing. Never allow anyone to make you feel guilty for using appropriate medicines or consulting trained physicians. Doing so is not a statement of doubt about God's healing power.

TROPHIMUS

Trophimus is another, lesser known, biblical example of illness. Trophimus was an associate of Paul, and 2 Timothy 4:20 reports that on one occasion Paul left Tromphius behind because he was sick. Why didn't Paul just heal Trophimus and continue the journey? Can we conclude that God must have wanted Tromphius to be ill? No, because the context indicates that Paul left Trophimus behind at Miletus because he was simply exhausted. The word translated *sick* in this passage can be translated *worn out*. When we overextend ourselves, we can suffer a host of physical problems, and that appears to be what happened in this case. Trophimus becoming exhausted is not an indication that God wants people to be ill.

EPAPHRODITUS

In Philippians 2:26–27, Paul mentions that Epaphroditus, a trusted assistant, was ill. But almost immediately Paul adds that God had mercy on him. The text reads, "For he longs for all of you and is distressed because you heard he was ill. Indeed he was ill, and almost died. But God had mercy on him, and not on him only but also on me, to spare me sorrow upon sorrow." The foundation for healing is mercy. The illness of Epaphroditus does not indicate that God wills for people to be sick but that he makes them well.

OUR LOVED ONES

We've considered a number of biblical examples of illness, but for most people, this issue is a personal one. The real question is not "What about Job?" or "What about Timothy?" but "What about my son, my mother, or my wife?" Each of us probably knows people who battled illness and did not get well. That's heartbreaking for us. It causes us to ask this question on a personal level. "What about my loved ones?" we wonder. "Did God want them to be sick? To die?"

We must remind ourselves that God is a God of mercy. He is a God who loves us and desires to give us good things. The story of Job shows that. Paul's experience confirms that, as does the report of Epaphroditus. God wants us to be well, and it will always be disappointing when some are not healed.

I have suffered illness myself. In fact, in the midst of a study on healing, I experienced pain in my back. A CAT scan revealed that I'd suffered a ruptured disc. I have wondered about these very questions myself—Why doesn't God heal me? Does he want me to suffer?

My experience along with the study of Scripture has taught me that just because God doesn't make me well doesn't mean that he is the source of my illness. I have also discovered that I do not need to defend God, as if he needs a public relations agent. I have long since gotten past that. Now I say, "God, I don't understand everything. It's a mystery to me. But I press on because of your compassion."

We continue to pray for those who are ill, and we continue to believe that God desires their healing. But for now, we admit that we do not know everything there is to know about God's grace, and we do not know everything about why some people are not healed or are not healed immediately. Remember Jesus' encounter with a blind man in John 9:1–3. The disciples asked Jesus who had sinned, the man or his parents, that caused him to be born blind. They wrongly assumed that the blindness was God's doing. In reality, the illness, although brought on by the Enemy, became an occasion for God's power to be demonstrated through healing, which brought glory to God.

We may never know why some people are not healed, but we do know this: Our God is a God of love, mercy, and compassion. And when we suffer, it is an occasion for his glory to be made known.

LET'S PRAY

Father—

Thank you for the gift of life. I ask that you will help me to treasure this earthly life, while it lasts, and to prepare myself for eternity with you. I long for this life to last forever, yet I know that is not your plan. I rejoice over my friends, my family, and the treasured relationships that I now enjoy. And I rejoice over the thought of being reunited with loved ones in heaven. You are the giver of life, and I worship you.

In Jesus' name,

Amen.

For small group discussion questions on this chapter and additional resources on healing, visit www.wesleyan.org/gsh.

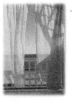

PART THREE

EXPERIENCING
HEALING

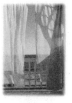

ELEVEN

How Can I Release God's Healing in My Life?

*Receiving and giving forgiveness is the first step to
unleashing God's power in our lives.*

"Is there any way I can avoid her?" Lynn thought as
she spotted Jamie walking toward her in the grocery store.
"All she ever does is complain."

Soon after Jamie's car accident, Lynn had felt
compassion for her, but after two months of hearing
incessant complaints about backaches, Lynn simply
avoided Jamie.

But before Lynn could turn into another aisle, Jamie spotted her. Surprisingly, she was all smiles and seemed to have a bounce in her step.

"Lynn!" Jamie called out, "You won't believe what happened. My back has been healed."

"Wow! I'm so glad to hear that," said Lynn. " Your chiropractor must be really great."

"It wasn't the chiropractor; it was God—definitely all God. He healed me."

Lynn looked puzzled.

"It was amazing," Jamie continued. " The other night some people came to my house to pray for healing. At one point, someone asked me if I was dealing with any spiritual issues in my life. I realized that I've really been bitter toward the driver who rear-ended me."

"So what happened?" Lynn asked.

" I went home, wrote him a letter. I told him that I forgave him for what had happened. The next day, my prayer group came again—and the pain went away."

"That's great," Lynn said, blinking away tears. "It's so great to see you smiling again."

If God wants us to be well, then why is anyone sick? That's a fair question. Certainly, God the Father is able to do anything he chooses to do. If he can part the Red Sea, still the storm, and raise Jesus from the dead, certainly he can cure cancer or diabetes or AIDS. Why doesn't he do that in every case?

I've discovered that while God always wants us to be well (he is a loving Heavenly Father), there are a number of reasons why people are not healed or are not healed immediately. In nearly every case, those reasons (I call them *blockages*) are often things that are under our control. Remember how God works in our lives. He works in us as we respond to his will. So there are a number of ways in which divine healing can be affected by our actions and attitudes. Once we clear away the blockage or blockages, whatever they may be, we place ourselves in a better position to receive God's gift of healing.

By the way, I'm not talking here about laws, things that always work in exactly the same way—such as the law of gravity. What goes up *always* comes down. It's a law that cannot fail. What I'm talking about here are principles. These are guidelines that show us the ways in which God usually works. These principles are not a guarantee of healing; but when we live by them, we are much more likely to experience the healing that God offers.

The first of these blockages has to do with our ability to recognize our need for inner healing that must precede physical healing. I first heard this from John Wimber. He and others who prayed for the sick had learned this important principle: we must be healed in spirit before we can be healed in body. And that spiritual healing depends upon giving and receiving forgiveness.

Spiritual before Physical

What do we mean by the term *inner healing*? Inner healing refers to our need to be healed from unresolved conflict in the heart, generally centering on unforgiveness, resentment, or bitterness. A second area of conflict has to do with our sexuality. Inner healing often is needed in a case where inappropriate sexual activity has been done either by us or to us. Some examples of that are adultery, rape, and molestation. These experiences create a broken, wounded inner spirit, especially for those who are victimized by them. Experience shows that the wounded spirit often needs to be healed before physical healing can take place.

Jesus sometimes dealt with spiritual issues before dealing with a physical one. An example is found in Luke 5:20, which records an incident in which people brought a man to Jesus for healing. The record states, "When Jesus saw their faith, he said, 'Friend, your sins are forgiven.'" Remember that the man had not been brought to Jesus for forgiveness. He was a paralytic. He was brought to Jesus because he couldn't walk and needed to be healed. But Jesus didn't start with the need for physical healing. He began dealing with the man in the spiritual domain and only later moved into the physical realm, healing the man's legs. Jesus focused on the spiritual, inner issue first and dealt with the physical problem later.

> Inner healing nearly always precedes physical healing.

Another example of how spiritual needs affect physical healing is found in Luke 9:42, which records an incident in which Jesus healed a young boy. The Bible says, "Even while the boy was coming, the demon threw him to the ground in a convulsion. But Jesus rebuked the evil spirit, healed the boy and gave him back to his father." In this case Jesus saw that the boy needed deliverance from demon possession as well as physical healing. Again Jesus chose to deal with the spiritual issue—deliverance—before the physical one. Jesus first rebuked the evil spirit, then healed the boy. Spiritual healing again preceded physical healing.

The first key to releasing God's healing power in our lives is to clear away our need for spiritual healing. Often that will center on the issue of giving and receiving forgiveness.

THE POWER OF UNCONFESSED SIN

We have all been tainted by sin. That sin, whether it is sin we have committed or a sinful act that was inflicted upon us by others, needs to be forgiven. We need forgiveness for the sins we commit, and we need to forgive others for wrongs they have done to us. When we do not give and receive forgiveness, our lives become filled with bitterness. We become wounded people. That is especially true when the sin involved has to do with our sexuality.

What this means is that when we come to God for physical healing, we appear to him as if we're in need of some spiritual help—and we are! Naturally, God wants to deal with our spiritual needs first. They are far deeper and ultimately more important than our physical condition. So as the Holy Spirit begins to put us back together, the first place that he applies his healing power is to our spirit. He heals our inner needs.

That is why unforgiveness creates a blockage for physical healing. Where there is unforgiveness, there can be no inner healing. And where there is no inner healing, there can be no physical healing. Unforgiveness is like a wall. When it goes up, it harbors Enemy activity on the inside and prevents the Holy Spirit from gaining access to the heart. To receive the gift of physical healing, it is essential to give and receive forgiveness, tearing down the wall that prevents the Spirit from working within us.

The Greater Power of Forgiveness

If unforgiveness is a wall, forgiveness is a wrecking ball. It knocks down the barrier to the Spirit's work. When that happens, demonic activity has no place to reside in our lives. We become open to God's work, including his healing power.

Here's an example of that. In 1983 I began to seriously investigate the matter of divine healing, and I spent some time around people who understood it far better than I did. I listened to them and observed their practice of divine healing. On one occasion, I was with some people who were praying for a young man who was demonized. There were about a dozen people praying for him. He was the most severely demonically affected person I have ever seen and displayed some bizarre and gross outward manifestations. We prayed and prayed, but it seemed that we weren't making much headway. I was a novice, of course, just trying to participate in what the others were doing.

After some time, someone suggested calling a young lady named Becky who was experienced in dealing with demonically afflicted people. Becky walked into the room and said, "Everybody sit down and be quiet." We did. She asked, "How long have you been praying?" We told her it had been about two hours. "What has happened?" she asked. We were embarrassed to admit that the man's condition had gotten worse.

Becky looked at the man, who was in obvious agony, and said to him, "There's no way these demons can stand against the power of Jesus unless there is some kind of fortress in your life that is permitting it." Then she did something that surprised us: she told all of us to go home. To the man who was demonized, she said, "Go home and think of any arenas of unforgiveness or impurity in your life that could be allowing the demonic activity to occupy you like this. Let God show you. Let him talk to you. And if he reveals some sin to you, confess it and ask for forgiveness. Then come back, and we'll take care of this problem."

The next day, the man returned and was set free after only a few moments of prayer. "What happened to you?" I asked him. "What went on during your prayer time that allowed Becky to so easily pray for you this morning?" He openly related his story to me. He had discovered unconfessed sin in his heart and had sought God's forgiveness. In fact, he had made several phone calls to ask forgiveness of people he had wronged. That act of confession had cleared the way for his spiritual healing.

As we purify our hearts, clearing away unconfessed sin, bitterness, and resentment, we remove all hiding places for the Enemy. When there is no fortress, no place for the Enemy to gain a foothold in our lives, we are fully available to the Holy Spirit. And when we are completely open to the Spirit, we can be healed. Spiritual healing tends to precede physical healing. That is why the giving and receiving of forgiveness is essential to receiving the gift of God's healing.

Giving and Receiving Forgiveness

Here's the key to all of this. There are two steps: one is to receive forgiveness, and the other is to give it. Let's talk about receiving forgiveness first. When you receive God's forgiveness, it produces wholeness in your life. We are broken people, but we are on a journey of receiving healing—healing that is ours in Christ Jesus.

Scripture declares our freedom from sin in Revelation 12:10: "Then I heard a loud voice in heaven say: 'Now have come the salvation and the power and the kingdom of our God, and the authority of his Christ. For the accuser of our brothers, who accuses them before our God day and night, has been hurled down.'"

It is true that the Enemy still goes around the land seeking whom he may devour, but the fact is the battle is already won. At the cross of Jesus Christ, Satan was consigned to death row. He knows that his destruction is coming. You now have the power of

> Unconfessed sin blocks our access to God's power, including his power to heal.

Christ within you to reject the accusations of the Enemy. You can be forgiven for your sin, by faith in Jesus Christ. When you receive that forgiveness, it releases God's power in you.

The second step in this process is to forgive others. On one occasion Jesus told a parable about a servant who did not forgive a debt and was severely punished. Jesus said, "This is how my heavenly

Father will treat each of you unless you forgive your brother in your heart" (Matt. 18:35). In the Sermon on the Mount, Jesus taught us how to pray. In his model prayer, the Lord's Prayer, Jesus taught us to pray, saying, "Forgive us our debts as we forgive our debtors." Then, in the very next verse, Jesus said, "For if you forgive men when they sin against you, your heavenly Father will also forgive you. But if you do not forgive men their sins, your Father will not forgive your sins" (Matt. 6:14–15).

Here's the issue: we must forgive others in order to release God's power in our lives. Inner healing precedes physical healing. Does that mean that every time a person isn't healed the reason is that they have unconfessed sin in or have not forgiven others? No, not at all. There can be many reasons why a person is not healed. But it is a clear principle in Scripture that inner healing precedes physical healing.

Have you fully received the inner healing that is yours?

DECLARING OUR IDENTITY

When we examine our hearts for unconfessed sin or the need to offer forgiveness to others, we remove a blockage to God's healing—a blockage or wall behind which the Enemy can hide. Yet it would be a mistake to become obsessed with demons and their presence in our lives. We center our thoughts on Christ, not on the Enemy.

Remember that when Jesus sent out the seventy-two in Luke 10, he sent them out to cast out demons and heal the sick. They did exactly that. When they returned, these disciples were elated that they had power over the Enemy. Jesus replied to them, "However, do not rejoice that the spirits submit to you, but rejoice that your names are written in heaven" (Luke 10:20). In other words, Jesus was saying, "Don't get excited about your power over demons—get excited about your identity as children of God!" Our relationship with Christ must be the focus of our spiritual lives. It would be a mistake to get preoccupied with the work of the Enemy.

So begin to clear the path to God's healing by examining your heart. Ask God to reveal any unconfessed sin. Examine yourself for bitterness, anger, or the need to offer forgiveness to others. Strengthen your relationship with God through Jesus Christ. Allow that relationship to be the epicenter of your prayer for healing. You are a child of God, by faith in Jesus Christ. As such, you are in a position to receive the gift of God's healing.

LET'S PRAY

Father—

To be healthy is one of the greatest desires of my heart. I know that you are the giver of life, and I believe that you can release your healing power in my life at any time. I ask you to do so now. I praise you for your goodness, compassion, and mercy. I thank you for the gift of life.

In Jesus' name I pray,

Amen.

For small group discussion questions on this chapter and additional resources on healing, visit www.wesleyan.org/gsh.

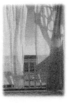

TWELVE

IS IT TRUE
THAT SIN
CAUSES DISEASE?

Some diseases are directly attributable to sins done by us,
and to the fact that we live in a sinful world.

As soon as Thomas walked through the office door, Tim
knew something was wrong. They had been accountability
partners for two years, and Tim always knew when his friend
had something on his mind.

"Bad news," Thomas said, his voice shaking.

"What's up?" Tim said, his mind racing through possible
scenarios for what Thomas would share.

"I just got some test results. I'm HIV positive."

Tim was flabbergasted. "You're what? But how? That's impossible."

"No, it is possible. A few years ago, I really messed up . . ." Thomas began to cry.

The two men sat in silence for a few minutes, neither knowing what to say.

Finally, Tim spoke. "I think a good place to begin is with confession. Let's talk about what happened."

"You're right," Thomas said slowly. "I've kept this to myself far too long."

L et's begin with a very strong disclaimer. As we discuss the connection between sin and illness, we *cannot* make a direct connection between sin and illness in most cases. For example, we would never say to someone for whom we were praying, "The reason you are ill is because you have sinned," or, "You are sick because of some sin in your life." To do so would be cruel and un-Christlike. There are many reasons why a person may not receive divine healing or may not receive it immediately. We do not assume that sin is the direct cause of illness in any individual case.

Yet it is true that there is a connection between sin and illness, and, therefore, between confession and healing. Let's look at what the Bible says.

THE CONNECTION BETWEEN SIN AND ILLNESS

Many people are hesitant to make a connection between sin and illness, but it is scriptural. The Bible says, "The LORD will send forth fearful plagues on you and your descendents. Harsh and prolong disasters and severe and lingering illnesses" (Deut. 28:59). What were the reasons for that pronouncement? It's stated in the latter verses of

Deuteronomy 28: "Because you did not obey the Lord your God" (Deut. 28:62). There are consequences for ignoring God's will in our lives, and one of those consequences can be illness. Let's examine several Scripture passages that make this point.

1 CORINTHIANS 11:29–30

Someone may object that the connection between sin and illness is seen only in the Old Testament. Yet the New Testament makes the connection as well. 1 Corinthians 11:29–30 states, "For all who eat and drink without discerning the body, eat and drink judgment against themselves. For this reason many of you are weak and ill, and some have died" (NRSV). Paul drew a clear connection between sin in the church—in this case, being flippant about the Lord's Supper—and illness, even death. In other words, people have violated God's ways, and they have brought death upon themselves as a result.

> In some cases, disease is a direct result of sinful choices.

JOHN 5

John 5 contains the account of Jesus' healing of a man who had been a paralytic for thirty-eight years. Some time after healing the man, Jesus said to him, "See, you are well again. Stop sinning or something worse may happen to you" (John 5:14). Although sin was not the cause of the man's paralysis, Jesus used the occasion to emphasize the cause-and-effect relationship between sin and illness. Two other passages make the same point. Psalm 107:17 says, "Some became fools through their rebellious ways and suffered afflictions because of their iniquities." Proverbs 3:7–8 states, "Do not be wise in your own eyes; fear the LORD and shun evil. This will bring health to your body and nourishment to your bones."

MATTHEW 18

In Matthew 18 a king is in dialogue with a servant who owes him a lot of money—the equivalent of millions of dollars in today's currency. Although the king generously forgives the man's debt, the servant later goes out and threatens to imprison a fellow servant who owes him what today would only be a few dollars. When the king hears of this, he is furious. In a rage, he orders the ungrateful servant to be thrown into jail and tortured. The parable ends with these words: "This is how my heavenly Father will treat each of you unless you forgive your brother from your heart" (Matt. 18:35). We see here an indication of the tremendous trauma we do to ourselves spiritually if we do not forgive one another. The power of sin—unforgiveness in this case—brings consequences that are both spiritual and physical.

HOLISTIC HEALING

We may be reluctant to admit the link between sin and illness because our Western minds are trained to separate the spiritual and physical worlds. In our way of thinking, the realm of the spirit has nothing at all to do with the physical world. But the Bible presents a different view. In Scripture, there is always a connection between the spiritual and physical worlds. If there is a problem in one, it affects the others. That's also true in people because we're spiritual creatures. Our physical, mental, emotional, and spiritual well-being is intertwined. Any problem in one area will affect the others.

> Human beings are holistic—the body, mind, and spirit affect one another.

The word *holistic* is often equated with a worldview that is virtually New Age. Yet the word itself, in this context, merely indicates the integration of body, mind, and spirit. That's an entirely biblical concept. When you have a problem in one area of your life, it affects the others. Physical problems often produce an emotional result, like depression. Emotional problems can produce a physical manifestation. For example, people who are under emotional stress often suffer physical symptoms such as stomach ulcers. And spiritual problems affect us physically and emotionally. We are whole beings.

Remember the case of King David, who committed adultery with Bathsheba and then arranged the murder of her husband, Uriah, in order to prevent the sin from becoming known. But David's sin was revealed, and he suffered terribly because of it.

In Psalm 51:12, David writes, "Restore to me the joy . . ." His sin produced an emotional result. In Psalm 31, David goes further in describing his physical and emotional pain, caused by sin: "Be merciful to me, O LORD, for I am in distress; my eyes grow weak with sorrow, my soul and my body with grief. My life is consumed by anguish and my years by groaning; my strength fails because of my affliction, and my bones grow weak" (Ps. 31:9–10).

The Bible makes the connection between sin and illness explicit. And, if we are honest with ourselves, we know that it is real. In some cases it is painfully obvious that sin results in illness. Some sexual sins carry the risk of disease. Some people are ill because they abuse alcohol, tobacco, drugs, or are obese. Some sins produce very clear physical results. Yet even when the connection is not so clear, there is still a connection between sin and illness. The damage that we inflict upon ourselves by disregarding God's commands is not limited to the spiritual realm. We may become physically ill as a result of sin.

CONFESSION AS CURE

If sin can produce illness, then what is the cure? It is confession. We've already seen that inner healing must precede physical healing. In the case of one who has sinned, that healing is brought about by confession.

What is confession? It is when we cease covering up our sin and expose it before God. Confession is when we stop justifying ourselves and agree with God that we have done wrong. Confession is being honest with God and ourselves about the true state of our souls.

In Psalm 51:3, David writes, "I know my transgressions." That is confession. In the original language, it was unnecessary for David to use the word *I*. It was understood from the context that the writer, David, was the subject of the verb *know*. Yet David chose to use the word, intensifying the statement. "I—yes, I—know my sin." He was deeply sorry for what he had done. That statement of confession is vital for experiencing God's healing power. Sin can be a root cause of illness. Confession releases God's grace into our lives, removing the offense of our sin. When we confess, we become candidates for healing—spiritually and physically.

SIN IN THE LIFE OF THOSE PRAYING

Sin can cause illness in an individual. It can also be a blockage of God's healing power if it exists *in those praying* for the sick person. James 5:16 says, "Therefore confess your sins to each other and pray for each other so that you may be healed. The prayer of a righteous man is powerful and effective." One of the prior verses states, "Is any one of you sick? He should call the elders of the church to pray over him and anoint him with oil in the name of the Lord" (James 5:14). Notice the order indicated: first, confess your sins to each other, then pray for each other that you may be healed. Those who pray for healing must also be in a right relationship with God in order to experience God's healing power.

I've seen that principle at work in my own ministry. On one occasion, two people in our congregation were miraculously healed. One had been suffering a loss of hearing; the other had a tumor in the throat. As church members gathered to pray for them, we began by confessing our own sins. Nobody was showboating their humility, but we prayed corporately, "Father, we confess that there are times that we do not measure up to the standard that you have for us, and we want to be that kind of people who do. We confess our sins to you. We know our sin, and we ask you to forgive us and cleanse us by the blood of Jesus." Thankfully, both people for whom we prayed were divinely healed.

It is important to restate that I do *not* believe that all sick people are ill because they have sinned. There are many blockages to healing. Sin in the life of the diseased person is one possible cause—but not necessarily the probable cause. There could be a number of other reasons. If sin is a factor, allow the Spirit of God to gently and tenderly bring conviction. Sometimes it is most appropriate to confess sin in a private, confidential setting, but sin must be confessed to release healing. It is the prayer of a *righteous* person that is powerful and effective—that is, of a person who is in a right standing before God.

Let us confess our sins so that we may be healed.

LET'S PRAY

Father—

I confess my sin before you. I have done wrong. I have thought wicked thoughts. I have offended both you and others. I am sorry, and I renounce my sinful ways. More than anything else, I want to live in a close, pure relationship with you. I ask for the forgiveness that you have promised in Jesus' name.

Amen.

For small group discussion questions on this chapter and additional resources on healing, visit www.wesleyan.org/gsh.

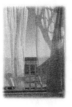

WHERE DO I NEED TO GO FOR HEALING?

*Healing comes when there is proper alignment
within the body of Christ.*

*Eastside Fellowship had seen better days. In five years
the congregation had dwindled from nearly three hundred
people to around eighty. Most of those who remained were
unsure how much longer the church could remain open. At a
Wednesday evening prayer meeting, Al Conner voiced what
many others had been thinking.*

*"Grace Tabernacle is killing us," Al whined. "They've
stolen six families from us in the last year."*

"Maybe they'd have stayed if we had given them a reason," Cora Albert answered.

"What's that supposed to mean?" Al asked.

"Nothing against our pastor," Ernie Hernandez chimed in, "but the preaching—well, let's say I've heard better."

Fifteen minutes later the group was still at it, alternately complaining about their pastor, the dearth of volunteers, declining attendance, and the megachurch across town.

Glenn Rhoades had been sitting silently on the third row. He stood slowly, then faced the group. "I think it's time to pray," he said. "For healing."

"Whatsa matter?" Ernie asked. "You sick or something?"

"Not for me," Glenn said. "For this church. For this community. For our families. For all of us. It's time we were healed."

Al and Ernie exchanged puzzled looks. "What's that supposed to mean?"

What is the institution in our culture that is most neglected today? Some would say marriage, and certainly marriage has suffered in our society in recent decades. Others might speak more broadly about the institution of the family. And the family has been under attack. Others might say education or government. Yet the most neglected—even abused—institution in our culture today is the church.

Consider the past two thousand years of history, and it is amazing that the church even exists. Think of the number of people who have been martyred for their faith and the number that are still being persecuted. Think of the church buildings that have been sacked and burned through the centuries. Also, remember that the church is neglected by those within it as often as it is abused by those on the outside. As discussed extensively in my book *God and His People,* infighting, apathy, and dissension have plagued the church over the centuries. Consider the forces that have opposed the institution of the church, and you will realize that it is incredible that the church continues to exist.

The church exists because it has a divine purpose. It is God's house of healing for those who dwell within. It is the church — not the family, not education, not government, not even health care — that brings wholeness to people. We find healing when we are in fellowship with God's people in the church. There is a trend today among many Christians to attend worship services only occasionally or not at all. That is a great mistake. When Christians make themselves absent from worship, they are removing themselves from the very community that brings healing.

CHURCH UNITY AND DIVINE HEALING

A healthy church brings health to those within it. Psalm 133:1–2 states, "How good and how pleasant it is when brothers live together in unity! It is like precious oil poured on the head, running down on the beard." Those verses are a description of the church, and it is a picture of harmony and health.

> God pours his blessings on a unified church. Healing is one of God's blessings.

In the Old Testament, oil is a symbol of God's presence. That's why people were anointed with oil. The substance itself did not have any special properties; it was used to acknowledge dependence upon God. These particular verses refer to an event recorded in Exodus 29, when Aaron, the brother of Moses, was consecrated as a priest. The image is of the Spirit of God flowing down over Aaron like oil. So Psalm 133 is telling us that when the church is unified, the Spirit of God flows down over it, as it did upon Aaron at the time of his consecration. Notice also that the flow of God's presence begins at the head, then moves through the whole body.

Psalm 133:3 adds another image to this picture: "It is as if the dew of Hermon were falling on Mount Zion." Mount Hermon is a large mountain, snowcapped most of the year. The climate of the Holy Land is very dry, with little rainfall. You can imagine how refreshing the runoff from that mountain would be—clear water flowing down to refresh the valley. And what is Mount Zion? In a literal sense, that refers to Jerusalem. We know from Scripture, however, that Mount Zion refers also to the church.

This is how the Psalm concludes: "For there the LORD bestows his blessing, even life forevermore." Here is the connection to health and healing. For when God's people—the church—dwell together in unity, it brings the presence of God's Spirit and wonderful blessings, specifically life.

In other words, the health of your church has a direct impact upon your personal health. When your church is healthy—that is, unified—that health splashes over onto the individuals within it. When the church dwells in unity, God blesses. Unity within the church is a starting point for divine healing. The church becomes the greenhouse, the venue in which health is released into our bodies. That means the church is the place to be in order to experience divine healing. If we want to experience the blessings that God has for us, we need to be among his people.

SIGNS OF CHURCH HEALTH

If the church is to be a house of healing, then it must first be a healthy, functional church. Unity is the key to church health, so if we are to experience wholeness as individuals and as a group, we need to discover something about unity. What does it look like when a church dwells in unity? How do we achieve unity as a church and, therefore, experience God's healing?

Here are the indicators of a greenhouse church—one that gives life to its members.

LOVE

The words "love one another" occur twelve times in Scripture, eight times in the present tense. That means we're to love one another habitually, as a way of life. This kind of love is not a feeling; it is an act of the will. We love our brothers and sisters in Christ not because they happen to be great people but because we have chosen to love them. First John 4:12 says, "No one has ever seen God; but if we love one another, God lives in us and his love is made complete in us." A healthy church is one in which the people love one another.

FELLOWSHIP

Paul compared the church to a human body, saying that we all belong to each other. If one is hurt, all suffer. If one rejoices, all rejoice. Being part of a healthy church is like having lots of caring brothers and sisters. It is a network of support.

FORBEARANCE

To forbear means to hold up, and, again, in Scripture it is mostly used in the present tense. The meaning is that we should constantly hold each other up. That doesn't mean we simply put up with each other. Instead, it means that we are understanding of each other's weaknesses and still love one another. Sometimes this word is translated *longsuffering*. That doesn't mean that we suffer a long time, but that we continually hold one another up in love and prayer in spite of our flaws and weaknesses.

CORRECTION

To correct is to instruct or admonish someone with encouragement. That is a delicate task, and difficult to do. No one likes to receive correction. But when we do, we grow. The whole church is made healthier when we hold each other accountable. If I am in an environment where someone corrects me, I know that I'm in a loving place.

WELCOME

When the church began on the day of Pentecost, the number of believers grew from 120 to 3,120 in a matter of hours. That was a huge influx of people. And not all of them were Jewish, as Christ's first disciples were. Very early in its history, the church had to make a place for those who were ethnically and culturally different from the majority. That made for some challenging times, but the church rose to the occasion, welcoming all who would come to Christ. A healthy church is a welcoming church.

> A healthy church is like a greenhouse; it's a place where people thrive.

HARMONY

To be in harmony is to be of the same mind. Do we have differences? Of course we do— lots of them. But we all believe in the same Lord, Jesus Christ. A healthy church is united in its focus on Christ.

CONFESSION

Scripture says that we are to confess our sins to one another. That's not a request; it's a command. It is much easier to confess sins to God than others, but we're commanded to do it. And, again, the command is given in the present tense. That means we are to do it habitually. A church in which members are willing to freely admit their faults is a healthy church.

PRAYER

James 5:16 urges us to pray specifically for healing. Prayer, in general, is the mark of a healthy church. In particular, prayer for healing is a sign of church health.

SUBMISSION

Healthy churches practice mutual submission. That means submitting to the will of others when necessary, regardless of age, gender, or social status. It means being willing to serve one another and learn from one another, to allow oneself to be corrected by others, regardless of who they are. We are enabled to achieve that level of humble submission as we are continuously filled with the Holy Spirit.

KINDNESS

In Ephesians 4:32, Paul advises us to be kind to one another, forgiving one another just as we are forgiven. It is always easy to give to someone when you expect something in return. Unconditional giving is something else, and that's the kindness that Paul talks about. It means to keep on forgiving one another, even when there is nothing given in return.

HOSPITALITY

In the ancient world, travel was extremely difficult. There were no luxury hotels or even motels. People stayed at inns, where they were available, and the accommodations were not good. That's why Christians were urged to practice hospitality. Caring for the needs of those who are traveling was an important spiritual exercise. Who are the strangers in our world? We are commanded to love them—that person next to you on the airplane, the one ahead of you in the checkout line, an immigrant to your community. Hospitality is opening your heart and your home to others. Healthy churches are hospitable places.

HUMILITY

Peter writes, "Clothe yourselves with humility toward one another" (1 Pet. 5:12). That's an interesting phrase, given the fact that Peter may have been recalling an event from the night before Jesus' crucifixion. Christ took off his outer garment and wrapped himself in a towel, then washed his disciples' feet. To be clothed with humility is to adopt the attitude that others are more important than oneself. It is the attitude that enables us to love and serve others, as Jesus served us. Healthy churches are filled with humble people.

SERVICE

Many people in the ancient world were slaves. So when the Bible tells us to serve one another, it is using strong language. The Apostle Paul didn't take it lightly when he advised people to be bond slaves to Jesus Christ. A bond slave was one who had gained the right to be free but chose to continue, willingly, in service to his or her master. The late Bill Bright of Campus Crusade for Christ was in the habit of signing his letters, "Bill Bright, a slave of Christ." That's a wonderful way of saying that he had given his life away to serve Christ. That attitude is the mark of a healthy Christian and a healthy church.

IN THE GREENHOUSE

When the church is healthy, it is like a greenhouse. It is a place of growth, life, and health for those inside. So being part of a healthy church fellowship is an important step toward receiving God's gift of healing. It is important to remember that the principles in this book are not laws. They are guidelines that indicate the usual ways in which God works and the things we can do to place ourselves in a position to receive his grace. So there is no guarantee that we can expect a miracle because we attend a good church. Yet God's house is a house of healing. When a church dwells in unity, the Holy Spirit will be present. And where the Spirit is present, there will be healing. Where can I go to experience God's healing? The best place to be is in the church.

LET'S PRAY

Father—

Thank you for the church. I am grateful for my brothers and sisters in Christ, who pray for me, encourage me, instruct me, and correct me. I pray that I may be useful to others as I serve you. Lord, help me to pray for others. I ask you now to have mercy on those in my fellowship who are ill. Touch them with your power, and make them whole.

In Jesus' name I ask this.

Amen.

For small group discussion questions on this chapter and additional resources on healing, visit www.wesleyan.org/gsh.

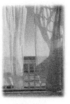

FOURTEEN

DO I HAVE ENOUGH FAITH TO BE HEALED?

If we are not receptive to God's power, we will not experience God's healing.

Sunlight streamed through the storefront of Paul Marks's convenience store. Not quite 6:00 on a June morning, Paul was busy making coffee and setting out donuts for the horde of customers that would soon invade his shop. Randy Cunningham emerged from the back room wearing a green Shop-A-Lot apron.

"Randy! Great to have you back."

"Yeah, I'm feeling a lot better." Randy seemed embarrassed to say the next words. "Um, thanks a lot for praying."

Paul nearly dropped a pot of fresh coffee. For several weeks, Randy had battled a respiratory infection. Paul's constant offers to pray for healing—even to anoint the younger man—had always been rebuffed. Paul laid a hand on Randy's shoulder.

"Glad to do it, man. I'm just glad you're feeling better . . . but I wasn't too sure you believed in the power of prayer."

"I didn't used to," Randy said flatly. "But I do now."

M any people have been wounded by inaccurate and insensitive statements made about the subject of faith and healing. On occasions when someone who was prayed for healing did not get well, I have heard those praying say, "You must lack faith." I can't think of a more insensitive statement to make to an ill person. I once heard a story about comments made at the graveside of a fine Christian man to the effect that he died because he lacked the faith that God could heal him. How cruel! Nearly all of the people for whom I have prayed genuinely believe that God is a loving Father and have an eager expectancy that he will release healing to them. There are a number of reasons why a person may not be divinely healed. To assume automatically that someone is ill because he or she lacks faith is dangerously wrong. Of all the issues surrounding the doctrine of divine healing, this one is perhaps the most overstated.

Yet the question remains: Is there a connection between faith and healing? The answer is unequivocally "Yes." I do not believe that lack of faith is *the* major blockage to experiencing healing; but it is one, and we need to address it.

The Faith of the Ill Person

It would be quite wrong to assume that lack of faith on the part of an ill person is the reason he or she is not made well. Yet Scripture indicates that the faith of those desiring healing has a direct bearing on whether or not God's healing power will be released. We need to understand the meaning of Scripture on this point for ourselves so we might gently direct others to put their full trust in our loving Father. Let's see what the Bible says about the relationship between faith and healing.

The Woman with a Hemorrhage

Luke records an incident in which a sick woman sought out Jesus for healing. She was hemorrhaging and had suffered from the problem for many years. Because there were so many people crowding around Jesus, the woman couldn't get to him directly. Believing that Jesus had the power to heal, she came up behind him and touched the edge of his cloak. Her bleeding stopped immediately.

Here's the interesting part! Jesus sensed that healing power had gone out from him, and he immediately asked who had touched him. When the woman identified herself, Jesus said,

> Our faith plays a part in the divine–human equation.

"Daughter your faith has healed you. Go in peace" (Luke 8:48). While it is not immediately apparent in the text of this story, it's interesting to note that in those days, various parts of some garments had a special meaning. The hem of a rabbi's garment symbolized, in the view of some, the Covenant—God's grand "contract" to love humanity. So the reason this woman touched the hem of Jesus' garment may have been that she saw the significance of the covenant between God and humankind, which includes the issue of healing. The bottom line is that Jesus used the occasion to emphasize the link between faith and healing.

THE IMPORTANCE OF FAITH

On one occasion, Jesus made this statement to his disciples. "If you believe, you will receive whatever you ask for in prayer" (Matt. 21:22). Jesus also said, "Have faith in God . . . I tell you the truth, if anyone says to this mountain, 'Go, throw yourself into the sea,' and does not doubt in his heart but believes that what he says will happen, it will be done for him" (Mark 11:22–23).

As you read these verses, you might wonder about times you prayed and did *not* see an answer to your prayer. That issue will be dealt with in later chapters. But for now, notice a key issue in these verses: there is great power in the act of faith.

THE NEED FOR FAITH

The converse is true also. Let's look at a negative example. When Jesus returned to his hometown of Nazareth, he was not well received. This is what Mark says about the incident: "[Jesus] could not do any miracles there, except lay his hands on a few sick people and heal them. And he was amazed at their lack of faith" (Mark 6:5–6). Where there is no faith, no miracles can take place.

> It would be a mistake to conclude that an individual's illness is caused by a lack of faith.

This means that faith is essential for divine healing. If we believe in God's goodness and his power—that is, if we believe that he is both willing and able to heal—then we can see more healing occur. When we do not believe that healing is possible, it will not take place.

However, we must be cautious. It would take a great leap of judgment to conclude that a lack of faith is the specific factor that has blocked healing in any given case. It is wrong to say to a diseased person, "If you had faith, you would be well." We simply don't make those judgments about people; there's no need to. Admittedly, lack of faith *can* be a blockage to healing. However, a person could have great faith and not be healed due to other factors blocking their healing.

God can and does heal, and we should encourage others to look expectantly to God for this gift. God still heals. When we believe that is true, we are in a better position to receive his healing power.

THE FAITH OF THOSE PRAYING

There is a second aspect to this connection between faith and healing, one that is often overlooked. If the need for faith on the part of the person in need of healing has sometimes been overemphasized, the need for faith on the part of the person praying for the healing of another person has perhaps been underemphasized. There is a connection between the faith of those praying and the release of God's healing power. That connection can be positive or negative. In at least one instance, we know that God's healing power was released on account of the faith of others—not of the diseased person. Lack of faith in those praying for the healing of another person can also be a blockage to God's healing power.

THE PARALYTIC

Luke 5 records the story of the paralytic who was brought to Jesus for healing by four friends. The house in which Jesus was teaching was so crowded that they couldn't get the man in the door, so they carried him up on the roof, cut a hole in the ceiling, and lowered the man down in front of Jesus. The Bible says, "When Jesus saw *their* faith, he said, 'Friend, your sins are forgiven,'" (Luke 5:20 emphasis added). A few moments later, Jesus healed the man. It's great to have friends who believe! Notice that the story never mentions the faith of the diseased man. It was the faith of those who brought him to Jesus that triggered a response. I believe that when God looks down from heaven and sees us praying in faith for the sick among us, he is greatly pleased. This incident shows that God responds to the faith displayed by those who pray for the sick.

A MODERN EXAMPLE

Years ago I was involved in a healing project with a medical doctor whom I'll call Aaron. Aaron told me about an account that he had witnessed involving a young lady who had been terribly injured in an automobile accident. Aaron wanted to organize prayer for the young woman, but she was in such desperate condition that it was difficult to find people who believed she could be healed. Finally Aaron gathered a group of students, all new Christians, to pray for the girl. Aaron admits that even his faith was weak in this case, because the girl's need was so great. But the students were convinced that God can do anything, and they "prayed up a storm." Here's how Aaron describes what happened next:

> I've never seen it before, and I've never seen it since. During our second round of prayer, I opened my eyes and saw the strangest sight on her skin. It looked like boiling oatmeal. It was just kind of bubbling. As a physician, I was interested in what was happening to the girl, and I watched this phenomenon move up her arm. My reaction was stunned silence, but one of the new believers with me was less intrigued. "Oh, that's gross!" she said, right in the middle of our prayer time.

And with tears in his eyes, Aaron went on to describe the healing power of God. The young woman was miraculously healed before his eyes.

Is that kind of thing common? Frankly, it is not. That is the only one like it that I've ever encountered, and I concede that this particular healing was quite bizarre. Yet it happened because the Father was pleased with the faith of those baby Christians and responded. The faithful prayer of righteous people avails much.

The Need for Faith

If the presence of faith is positive, its absence can be negative. Where there is no faith, miracles cannot occur. There have been times, not often, when I have been praying for healing and sensed that someone present had no confidence that God could heal. By a comment or by body language, that person revealed that they simply did not believe healing was possible. As gently as I could, I have gone to the person in question and tenderly and politely asked if they would be open to absenting themselves from the time of prayer. It is essential that those who pray for healing believe that healing is possible. God is thrilled by our faith, and he honors it. Yet where there is not faith, his healing power will not be released. That was the experience of Jesus himself when he returned to his hometown of Nazareth. Scripture tells us, "He could not do any miracles there, except lay his hands on a few sick people and heal them. And he was amazed at their lack of faith" (Mark 6:5–6).

Faith Enough

So how much faith do I need in order to pray for healing? How much faith do I need in order to be healed? How can I know that when there is some blockage to the release of God's healing power, my faith is not part of the problem?

Here is how much faith you need: enough to believe that God still heals. Jesus said that faith even the size of a mustard seed—just a tiny grain—is enough to move mountains. It is not the *amount* of faith that matters, but the release of whatever faith you do have. Do you believe that God still heals? Do you believe that God can heal you and those around you? That is faith enough. Trust God and receive his gift of healing.

LET'S PRAY

Father—

I feel like the man who prayed, "I do believe; help my unbelief." I believe that you are real, and I believe that you are good. Yet I struggle to believe that you will heal. I want greater faith, Lord. I am seeking you with my whole heart. Please hear my prayer and enable me to persevere in loving you and serving you.

In Jesus' name,

Amen.

For small group discussion questions on this chapter and additional resources on healing, visit www.wesleyan.org/gsh.

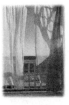

WHAT IS MY ROLE IN BRINGING HEALING?

When I reflect the likeness of God's Son,
I am a carrier of healing.

"You guys go ahead. I'll stay here and get some work done."

Norm Cook hated the idea of provoking a confrontation, but his wife always seemed to have work to do when their small group took on a prayer assignment. Last month she had discovered a pile of laundry as the team headed for the nursing home. This month the garden miraculously sprouted weeds on the day of Edie Johnsen's surgery.

"Honey, can't the gardening wait a day? I'd really like you to join us."

Louise heaved a sigh. "I know, but I have so much to do . . . and it seems like such a waste of time."

"Waste of time?"

"I'd like to support Edie. But honestly, I don't see how praying for her will make a difference at this point. I'd like to see our group do something useful."

"You mean a missions trip or something?"

"Yeah, some real work. Something Jesus would do. All we ever do is hold hands with sick people."

"I guess you're right," Norm said. "We do spend a lot of time praying for the sick." He paused. "But then, Jesus did too."

What does any of this have to do with me? That's a good question. Many people believe that God still heals but struggle to see how they fit into the picture. Are we all healers? Does everyone have a gift for healing? What role am I to play in God's healing work? We may not all be especially gifted as healers, but all of us are to become like Christ. After all, that's what the word *Christian* means—a follower of Christ. And as Christ's representatives, each of us will be involved in doing what he did. That will include healing.

MADE IN GOD'S IMAGE

The Bible tells us that human beings were made in the image of God—every one of us. Genesis records these words: "Then God said, 'Let us make man in our image, in our likeness, and let them rule. . . . So God created man in his own image, in the image of God he created him; male and female he created them" (Gen. 1:26, 27). A similar statement is made in Genesis 5:1, where the story of Noah begins. It says, "This is the written account of Adam's line. When God created man he made him in the likeness of God." The meaning in both places is that human beings were made to resemble their creator. We were crafted as copies of the original.

What does that mean? It means that God put us together in such a way that we would resemble him—not physically but morally. We would think, act, and respond as he did. In that sense, we are to be like God.

DAMAGED BY THE FALL

There was a problem, however. Human beings chose to ignore God's direction to them and to make their own choices. Adam and Eve enjoyed a perfect existence in the Garden of Eden, but they sinned. They disregarded God's instruction and incurred his penalty. Furthermore, that penalty affects all of us. The Apostle Paul puts it this way in Romans 3:23, "For all have sinned and fallen short of the glory of God." Adam and Eve were banished from the Garden because of their sin, and the world was placed under a curse. Every one of us lives under that curse today.

> When we think and act as Jesus did, we reflect the image of God.

Yet even after the Fall, Scripture refers to the fact that we are made in the likeness of God (see Gen. 5:1). Even in a world so broken that a brother, Cain, killed his own brother, Abel, we are still made in God's image. Broken and twisted though it is, we still bear the image of God in some way. That means that you are special. Even though you have failed God, even though you make many mistakes, even though your life may now be marked by sickness and suffering, you're still a person made in the image of God.

PERFECTLY REFLECTED IN CHRIST

Since we have been damaged by sin, God sent his son, Jesus, to give us a clear image of himself. In 2 Corinthians 4:4, Paul says that Christ is "the image of God." In Colossians 1:15 Paul says that Christ is "the image of this invisible God." Again, Paul writes in Colossians 1:19, "For God was pleased to have all his fullness dwell in him," and the writer of Hebrews says, that Jesus is "the radiance of God's glory, and the exact representation of his being" (Heb. 1:3).

Some 1,500 years later, Martin Luther commented that he didn't understand much about God, but when he looked at Jesus, he understood God better. Jesus came to restore all things, and he came to restore the image of God in you.

PERFECTLY RESTORED IN CHRIST

When we are united with Christ—a favorite expression of the Apostle Paul—the image of God is restored in us. When we think and act as Jesus did, we once again reflect the glory of God; we are like him. Scripture says that we have been made as a replica of God; we have his image stamped upon us. The brokenness in our world—and in you—stems from the fact that we have lost a part of the image of God; we no longer resemble him in the way he envisioned. Yet when we are united with Christ, that image is restored. Paul said in Romans 8:29 that we are to be "conformed to the likeness of his Son." In 2 Corinthians 3:18, he writes that we are "transformed into his likeness with ever-increasing glory." Colossians 3:9 states, "You have taken off your old self with its practices, and have put on the new self." Ephesians 4:24 tells us,

> As we become like Christ, we will develop great compassion for the sick.

"Put on the new self, created to be like God in true righteousness and holiness."

Scripture is clear on this point: when we are "in Christ," we are changed. We are transformed by the Spirit of God, and we come to resemble him. Does that mean that we are perfect, never make mistakes, and always respond precisely as Jesus would? No, it doesn't. We're still human beings, after all. Yet we gain power and understanding, and we gradually grow to become more and more like Jesus Christ. We begin to discover the true selves that God created us to be.

REFLECTING CHRIST

In John 5 Jesus describes the manner in which he reflects the Father's glory. Jesus said, "I tell you the truth, the Son can do nothing by himself; he can do only what he sees his Father doing, because whatever the Father does the Son also does." (John 5:19). In other words, Jesus mirrored the Father. That is a description of what it means to bear the image of God. When we reflect God's image, we do what he would do. So what does that mean for healing?

First, we know that Jesus was a healer. So as his followers — his imitators — we must be carriers of healing also. Jesus came to bring God's kingdom to earth. One sign of that Kingdom is healing. Jesus healed wherever he went, not as a kind of magic show or simply to display random acts of kindness but because he was establishing the reign of God. Wherever God's reign is established, there will be healing, so healing power accompanied Jesus everywhere. When we think and act as Jesus did, we will call upon God to release his healing power to those in need.

Second, we will be faithful to Christ by acting upon his commands. Jesus' final words on earth are recorded in Matthew 28:18–20, which says, "Then Jesus came to them and said, 'All authority in heaven and earth has been given to me. Therefore go and make disciples of all nations, baptizing them in the name of the Father and of the Son and of the Holy Spirit, and teaching them to obey everything I have commanded you. And surely I am with you always, to the very end of the age."

Jesus commissioned us to go into the world, continuing the ministry that he had begun. We are to continue to set things right, just as Jesus did, bringing hope, healing, and restoration to a world that has been broken by sin. When we reflect the image of Christ, we will be carriers of hope and healing, just as he was. And the promise that concludes our commission is vital. Christ is with us to the very end of the age, giving us the power and authority to put his words into action.

Remember that Jesus did nothing except what he saw the Father doing. As bearers of Christ's image, we will do what we have seen him doing. We will evangelize, lay hands on the sick and pray for them, and deliver people, setting them free from the power of darkness. What is our part in the ministry of healing? It is to be Christians—little Christs, as Martin Luther put it—reflecting the glory of God by bringing hope and healing to a broken world, just as Jesus did.

LET'S PRAY

Father—

I wish to be a carrier of your healing power. I have no power to heal, and I know it. Yet I see that healing follows wherever Jesus goes. As I follow him with my whole heart, let your healing power surround me. I pray that I may be an agent of healing and wholeness to those around me.

Let it be so, in Jesus' name,

Amen.

For small group discussion questions on this chapter and additional resources on healing, visit www.wesleyan.org/gsh.

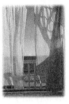

SIXTEEN

Do I Have the Spiritual Authority to Pray for Healing?

God has given the authority to heal to the church—
and, therefore, to believers.

Shauna James loved her new job—for the most part. But delivering flowers was sometimes depressing. Residential deliveries were always met with a smile, but much of the time Shauna's trips were to a hospital room or a funeral home.

As she looked over at the bouquet of yellow daisies with a "Get Well" card attached, Shauna sighed. She walked through the halls of the hospital looking for room 203, where she should find Stella Simmons. Expecting an older woman,

Shauna was surprised to find a young, twentysomething girl lying on the hospital bed.

"Umm, are you Stella Simmons?" Shauna asked as she entered the room.

"Yeah," Stella replied. It looked to Shauna as though the girl had been crying. "I'm sorry I'm so upset. I'm just sick of being in the hospital."

Shauna sensed that she should pray for the young woman, but she was unsure. Shauna was a new Christian, "I don't even know how to pray for healing," she thought.

Shauna set the bouquet on the nightstand and hesitated. "Oh well," she thought, "I believe in Jesus—that ought to be enough." She gripped Stella's hand.

"Would you mind if I pray for you?"

O ne of the blockages to the release of God's healing power is a lack of understanding of spiritual authority. Many people do not pray for healing—either for themselves or for others—because they simply don't think they can. They see themselves as spiritually weak or immature, not up to the Herculean task of praying people well. Perhaps you have had thoughts like, "I'd better call the pastor to pray about this," or, "I wish I had more faith so I could get God to hear my prayers." In reality, all believers have the spiritual authority to pray for healing.

THE EXERCISE OF SPIRITUAL AUTHORITY

Matthew 8 records the story of a Roman centurion who came to Jesus with a problem. A centurion was an officer who had charge of one hundred men. This centurion's servant was ill, so the man came to Jesus about the matter. As soon as Jesus heard that the servant was ill, he was ready to stop what he was doing, go to the nearby town where the boy lay ill, and heal him. But the centurion protested that the journey was unnecessary. He said, "Lord, I do not deserve to have you come under my roof. But just say the word and my servant will be healed. For I myself am a man under authority, with soldiers under me. I tell this one, 'Go,' and he goes; and that one, 'Come,' and he comes. I say to my servant, 'Do this,' and he does it" (Matt. 8:8–9). Jesus was so astonished by the man's faith that he healed the servant despite the distance.

This military man understood the principle of authority very well. He realized that when a person in authority speaks the word, that word will be accomplished.

When we operate in faith, we exercise authority. We do that by *speaking* the Word of God. God has given spiritual authority to various people at various times, and he has given the authority to heal to the church. Many people do not get well because they do not understand spiritual authority and do not exercise it—by speaking it.

> God has given spiritual authority to the church through Jesus Christ.

Here is a theology of healing in a nutshell. God's will is for healing. When we come into conformity with his will, we will speak and declare those things that align with his will and his Word.

As we speak God's Word, he watches over it to perform it (Jer. 1:12). Our prayers are sometimes requests, but at other times they are declarations, stating God's will through his Word over a situation. When we declare God's will, we function, as Paul Bilheimer puts it, as "enforcers" of heaven's will on earth. Thus, Jesus taught his followers to pray, "your kingdom come, your will be done *on earth* as it is in heaven" (Matt. 6:10, emphasis added). This is why God cares about our prayer life. He listens for us to pray his will, his Word. And when we do, he "backs it up." So as we face sickness and disease we declare God's will for healing. And God watches over that word. This is the foundation of our prayer for healing.

AUTHORITY IN THE COVENANT

In the beginning God gave authority to Adam and Eve. They were given charge over all of creation, according to Genesis 1:26. Adam and Eve were placed in the world and told to tend it—to have dominion over it. They had authority.

But Adam and Eve failed in their exercise of authority, and they lost that authority. As a result, the world came under the control of the Enemy. Charles Capps uses a football metaphor to describe what happened: Adam "fumbled the ball" and Satan "picked it up and ran with it." Adam and Eve should have said to Satan, "God gave us this planet. We have authority to be here. You do not. Therefore, based on the authority we have been given from God, we command you to leave." That would have been the last we heard of Satan, but that is not what happened.

> Rather than complain about illness, we should claim our authority in Christ and pray for healing.

Capps also uses terminology from the real estate business to describe this loss of authority, saying that although God owned the earth, he had "leased" it to Adam, giving him dominion over it. When Adam sinned, he placed himself under the authority of Satan, since one is a slave to the one to whom he submits. Romans 6:16 states, "Don't you know that when you offer yourselves to someone to obey him as slaves, you are slaves to the one whom you obey . . .?" Adam, according to Capps, "subleased" the earth to Satan, giving the Enemy control over the planet.

That left God, in a manner of speaking, on the outside looking in at his own creation. Yet because God always keeps his word, he would not simply take back control of the world. There needed to be some action by which God regained "legal" access to the world. Therefore, God formed a covenant with Abram. A covenant is an agreement between two parties that makes them one. Under the terms of a covenant, everything each party has belongs to the other. There are two types of covenant. A *parity covenant* is among equals—persons who have similar assets. A *suzerain covenant* is one between non-equals, such as a king and a slave. In a suzerain covenant, the king might state, "All the resources of my kingdom are at your disposal." The slave might respond, "What do I bring to this covenant? I have nothing." The king would reply, "I want the one thing you have— you and your descendents! I want your loyalty, your love."

When God made a covenant with Abram, it was a suzerain covenant. What God needed was Abram himself, and—because a covenant is binding upon future generations—Abram's descendents. This covenant set the stage for what would happen many years later to one of Abram's descendents, Mary. The Holy Spirit overshadowed Mary, and she conceived a child even though she had not had relations with a man.

Since Jesus was born of a human female, he was fully human. But since he was conceived by the Holy Spirit, Jesus was divine as well. Jesus' humanity gave him the "legal right" to be on planet earth. Remember, the earth had been turned over to humankind through Adam and Eve's "earth lease," as Capps has called it. Yet Jesus' divinity gave him moral superiority and authority over Satan, who controlled the whole human race.

At last, there was one person on the earth—Jesus—who was not under the authority of Satan. In a sense, a new human race had come to the earth through Jesus. That is why Jesus is sometimes called the "last Adam" (Rom. 5:15–17; 1 Cor. 15:45). God had given the earth to a human being (Adam means humankind). And that human being had released the planet to Satan. Since a human being (Adam) had given the earth away, only another human being (Jesus) could get it back. And this turns our focus to Jesus, who was fully human yet was divine, and therefore had moral authority.

The arrival of Jesus on planet earth sets the stage for the cosmic struggle between God and Satan. Jesus' ministry is focused on undoing, on destroying, the work of Satan (1 John 3:8). As we now know, Satan lost that battle, and Jesus won. (For a more complete discussion of this point, see my book *The Covenant*.)

AUTHORITY IN JESUS CHRIST

So where do we come in? Before he ascended into heaven, Jesus made this statement, "All authority in heaven and on earth has been given to me. Therefore go and make disciples . . ." (Matt. 28:18–19). Here is our place in the authority structure. Jesus has seized control of the world. And he has commissioned his followers to exercise that authority in his name. Remember that one of the primary reasons Jesus came was to bring healing. So when he commissioned his followers to go into the world and exercise authority in his name, Jesus intended for them to carry on the ministry of healing.

> God has given spiritual authority to the church through Jesus Christ.

How do we know that we have the spiritual authority to pray for and expect divine healing? We know that because Jesus has that authority, and he gave it to us. God has given the authority to heal to the church—and, therefore, to believers. We do not heal because we have power. We heal because God has power and we have been given the authority to release that power in Jesus' name.

THE EXERCISE OF SPIRITUAL AUTHORITY

Having authority is one thing; exercising that authority is something else. Probably all of us have seen examples of people who had authority but did not exercise it or exercised it poorly. For example, parents have authority by virtue of their position in the household, yet they do not always use that authority to provide for and discipline their children. In the same way, Christians have the authority to call for healing in Jesus' name, but we do not always exercise that authority.

CLAIMING AUTHORITY

Jesus said, "Have faith in God. . . . I tell you the truth, if anyone says to this mountain, 'Go, throw yourself into the sea,' and does not doubt in his heart but believes that what he says will happen, it will be done for him. Therefore I tell you, whatever you ask for in prayer, believe that you have received it, and it will be yours" (Mark 11:23–24). You might say, "Wait a minute! I've prayed for things before and did not receive them." It is within the framework of the Covenant that we may ask and receive from God. We may rightly call for, in the name of Jesus Christ, those things given to us through him.

Here's an example of that. When we are sick, we often spend a lot of energy complaining about our illness. Instead, we could say, "As a child of God and as one who is in covenant with Almighty God, I choose to receive the healing that is mine in Jesus' name." That is exercising authority. As children of God, we have the privilege of asking that the covenental power of God be exercised on our behalf.

EXERCISING FAITH

Exercising covenantal authority is an act of faith. Luke 17:3–6 says:

> "So watch yourselves. If your brother sins, rebuke him, and if he repents, forgive him. If he sins against you seven times in a day, and seven times comes back to you and says, 'I repent,' forgive him.'"
>
> The apostles said to the Lord, "Increase our faith!"
>
> He replied, "If you have faith as small as a mustard seed, you can say to this mulberry tree, 'Be uprooted and planted in the sea,' and it will obey you."

Jesus told his disciples that if they had faith the size of a tiny mustard seed, they could speak to a mulberry tree—which has an extensive root system—and command it to be uprooted. The disciples realized that Jesus was not talking about a tree removal service. He was talking about the root of bitterness that can grow in the human heart after having been wronged. When someone harms us, we can either let the root of bitterness take hold, digging itself deeper and deeper into the heart. Or, by the authority given to us by God, we can renounce that root of bitterness and command it to be gone from our lives. Jesus' response told his disciples that they didn't need more faith; they simply needed to exercise what little faith they did have by declaring that which is conformity with God's Word, God's will, and God's way.

The same is true for us. We are to exercise the authority given to us by *speaking* to sickness—coming against it with the authority we have in Christ.

LET'S PRAY

Father—

I choose to exercise the authority that you have given to me through Jesus Christ. I will no longer cower in the face of disease or pain, but I will pray boldly—even speaking to disease, commanding it to be gone, in accordance so that your healing power may be released to those who suffer.

I pray this in the name of Jesus,
Amen.

For small group discussion questions on this chapter and additional resources on healing, visit www.wesleyan.org/gsh.

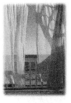

SEVENTEEN

How Does My Spiritual Life Affect My Prayers?

*Healing is enhanced by fasting, praying,
and seeing what the Father is doing.*

---

*"I've heard Pastor Brad say that we all have the authority
to heal, but I just don't believe it. I've asked God to heal lots of
people, and most of them died. I just don't have the gift."*

*Michael Benson sank a four-foot putt, then looked up at
his partner, Lionel Green. "What do you think?"*

*Lionel nodded. The two played eighteen holes together
most Saturday mornings, and Lionel knew a lot about his
partner from their meandering conversations on the fairway.*

He liked Michael but also realized that his friend's spiritual life was ineffective in many areas—not just prayer for healing.

"So what about you?" Michael asked. "Do you have the gift of healing?"

"I don't think that's my spiritual gift," Lionel said, "but I've definitely seen God work. I've seen people healed."

"Really?" Michael was surprised. "So why do you think your prayers are more effective than mine?"

"I don't know," Lionel demurred. "By the way, I haven't seen you at Bible study for a couple of months. Are you still reading the Word?"

"Oh, yeah," Michael said vaguely. "When I get time. I've been a little busy . . . Hey, I've got tickets to the Rams game on Sunday. Wanna go?"

When we pray for healing, we are operating within our covenant rights as children of God. So when we come to the Father in prayer, it is important that we are in a right relationship with him. We've already seen the connection between confession and healing. Unconfessed sin, bitterness, and resentment can be significant blockages to healing. Other aspects of spiritual life affect healing also. When they are in order, we will be more effective in praying for healing. When they are not as they should be, these areas of our spiritual life can be blockages to the release of God's healing power in our lives.

FASTING AND PRAYER

Mark 9 records an incident in which Jesus healed a boy who was demon possessed. It was a difficult case, and Jesus' disciples were unable to help the boy. In desperation, the boy's father explained the situation to Jesus who then cast the demon out of the boy. Later, when they were alone, the disciples asked Jesus why they were unable to cast out the demon. Jesus replied, "This kind can come out only by prayer" (Mark 9:29). Some translations say only "by prayer," but some of the early manuscripts of the Bible along with a number of modern translations say "prayer and fasting."

> There is a direct connection between our spiritual vitality and our ability to pray effectively.

What's intriguing about this incident is that the disciples did not ask Jesus to teach them when to pray or how to fast. They seemed to know *how* to do these things. The issue was that they needed to do them more often. These disciples had been traveling with Jesus for some time, and they must have known that he fasted and prayed often. Jesus was in the habit of getting up early to find some quiet place to pray. And he often would sneak off by himself to be alone in prayer. Jesus' instruction here simply told them that they needed to be doing the same thing.

It's interesting as well that on the other occasion when the disciples asked about prayer, they said, "Lord, teach us to pray" (Luke 11:1). They didn't say, "Teach us *how* to pray but" but "Teach us *to* pray"—to just do it! It isn't clear that the phrasing of that verse is intentional, but it is interesting. The disciples seemed to understand what prayer and fasting are all about. They just didn't spend enough time doing them.

There is a connection between our spiritual vitality and our ability to pray effectively for healing. When we are in tune with the Father through the spiritual disciplines of prayer and fasting, we will pray more effectively for healing. Again, this is a principle, not a law. The fact that we may fast before going to the hospital to pray for an ill person is not a guarantee that the person will be miraculously healed. But when we are in touch with the

Father, we are much more likely to pray effectively, and we are more likely to see healing take place.

SEEING WHAT THE FATHER IS DOING

Our spiritual connection goes beyond the disciplines of prayer and fasting. When we are most in tune with God, we will begin to know his heart and sense his intentions for us and those around us. We will see what the Father is doing and join him in it. When we are unable to see what the Father is doing, our prayers will be ineffective.

JESUS' EYES ON THE FATHER

John was the disciple who knew Jesus best. Of the Twelve, there was an inner circle of three: Peter, James, and John. Of those three, John is the one who is called "the disciple whom Jesus loved." Here is what John has to say about this very issue of seeing what the Father is doing.

John 5:19 says, "Jesus gave them this answer: 'I tell you the truth, the Son can do nothing by himself; he can do only what he sees the Father doing, because whatever the Father does the Son does also.'"

John 5:30 records these words of Christ: "By myself I can do nothing; I judge only as I hear, and my judgment is just, for I seek not to please myself but him who sent me." This is the second time Jesus says, "I can't do it on my own; I'm only doing what the Father tells me to do."

John 8:28 says, "So Jesus said, 'When you have lifted up the Son of Man, then you will know that I am the one I claim to be and that I do nothing on my own but speak just what the Father has taught me.'"

John 12:49 says, "For I did not speak of my accord, but the Father who sent me commanded me what to say and how to say it."

John 14:10 says, "Don't you believe that I am in the Father, and that the Father is in me? The words I say to you are not just my own. Rather, it is the Father, living in me, who is doing his work."

Clearly, Jesus understood this vital connection to the Father. Our Lord knew that he was about his Father's business. That should be true of every disciple of Christ, and it should be especially true as we look to extend Christ's ministry of healing. One of the ways to pray for the sick more effectively is to see what the Father is doing and join him in it.

LOOKING FOR THE FATHER'S WORK

How do we gain a sense of where God is working and what he wants us to do? Let the Holy Spirit put an impression on your heart. As you're praying for someone, he may show you something very important about how to deal with that person. On one occasion I was praying for the healing of a man, and I kept sensing a very strong impression of the word *brother-in-law*. I kept hearing it over and over in my mind, "Brother-in-law, brother-in-law." Finally I asked the man, "Is there anything about your brother-in-law that I ought to know?"

His eyes widened in surprise. He asked, "How did you know that?"

"I don't really know anything," I said. "I just sensed that I should ask you."

He then related the great bitterness he had in his heart toward his brother-in-law. "Let's take care of that first," I said, "and then take the matter of healing before the Lord." When you look for what the Father is doing, he will reveal needs to you.

A caution is in order here, because it can be terribly presumptuous to tell another person, "God told me to tell you . . ." Even from the pulpit, I am cautious about using the phrase, "God told me." I find it better to say things like, "God seems to be leading in this direction," or, "If I'm hearing the Father correctly . . ." We need to be careful about pronouncing to other people what we *think* God is doing, because we could be wrong.

Yet most of us are *too* cautious in this area. We are reluctant to follow the Spirit's leading, and we need greater boldness in respond-ing to what God lays upon our hearts. When Jesus healed people on the Sabbath, the religious leaders of the day became upset because they thought it was a violation of God's law to "work" on the Sabbath by heal-ing someone. But Jesus was bold about his calling to minister healing to people, and he asserted that he would keep right on doing it. He was in tune with the Father's will, and that gave him boldness to act on that will. The same will be true for us as we sense what the Father is doing.

> When we keep our eyes on the Father, we will see healing.

HEARING FROM GOD

Now how does one receive a word from the Lord? It comes in various forms. John Wimber taught that it might be visual, a picture that forms in the mind. Sometimes, he said, it may be more like a banner headline, a statement that is strongly impressed upon you by the Holy Spirit. For me personally, it comes as a very definite impres-sion—something that you simply know that you know.

My wife and I were praying for a married couple, and she started addressing an issue in prayer that I thought had no connection to the person for whom we were praying. She said, "Fear. The key word here is *fear*." Although we had prayed for this couple for some time, we had seen no change. But when we addressed the issue of fear in our prayers, things changed.

On other occasions, God may simply place his words in your mouth so that you literally speak them. In chapter 2, I related a time when I prayed for a song evangelist who was ill. I found words coming from my lips that I had never spoken before. I said, "I command this spirit to come out in the name of Jesus." I was stunned at myself. I was speaking the words God wanted me to speak.

The Importance of Purity

There is a sequence in Scripture that is very important, and it is illustrated in Jesus' cleansing of the Temple, recorded in Matthew 21:12–16.

> Jesus entered the temple area and drove out all who were buying and selling there. He overturned the tables of the money changers and the benches of those selling doves. "It is written," he said to them, " 'My house will be called a house of prayer,' but you are making it a 'den of robbers.'"
>
> The blind and the lame came to him at the temple, and he healed them. But when the chief priests and the teachers of the law saw the wonderful things he did and the children shouting in the temple area, "Hosanna to the Son of David," they were indignant.
>
> "Do you hear what these children are saying?" they asked him.
>
> "Yes," replied Jesus, "have you never read, "'From the lips of children and infants you have ordained praise'?"

Notice the sequence of events. First Jesus cleansed the Temple of impurity so that people could pray. Then Jesus established his presence in the Temple, and people came to him for healing. Finally, people shouted their praise to God for the wonderful things they had seen. Purity, prayer, presence, power, praise: that seems to be the biblical sequence. When we purify our hearts before God and cry out to him, we will experience his presence. With his presence comes his power. After the demonstration of power comes unrestrained praise. If our prayers for healing are ineffective, it might be because we are looking for God's power without first purifying ourselves and seeking his presence. But when we unite ourselves with the Father through fasting and prayer, then look and listen to discern his will, we place ourselves in a position to see the release of his healing power.

LET'S PRAY

Father—

Whenever I seek you, you reveal yourself to me. Yet I do not seek you consistently. I have allowed my work, my family, and the busyness of life to distract me from the one thing that matters most—my relationship with you. Lord, help me to be diligent in the care of my soul, feeding on Scripture and drawing strength from you through prayer. Make me a strong, healthy person so that I may minister health to those in need.

In Jesus' name I ask this.

Amen.

For small group discussion questions on this chapter and additional resources on healing, visit www.wesleyan.org/gsh.

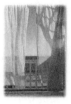

EIGHTEEN

IF I NEGLECT MY HEALTH, WHAT CAN I EXPECT FROM GOD?

*Our lifestyle can significantly affect our
ability to experience healing*

"Pastor, how come you never preach about healing?"

The question took Pastor Ron by surprise. After six years at Grace Church, he thought he had declared the "whole counsel of God."

"I'll be planning sermons for the next year during the summer," Ron said. "I'll see if God lays that subject on my heart."

Yet Ron already knew that he would not tackle the subject of divine healing. More than one hundred pounds overweight, the thirty-five-year-old pastor was experiencing several health problems directly related to obesity. His joints ached every time he walked more than a few yards, and he was short of breath when climbing stairs or mowing the lawn.

"Look at me," Ron thought dejectedly. "My blood pressure is out of control, and my cholesterol is off the chart. My life is a mess. How in the world could I preach about healing?"

Ron sank into his office chair and stared out the window. Then he reached for the jar of M&M's on the corner of his desk. "Worst of all," he thought, "I just can't quit eating."

I recently lost eighty pounds. I am not proud of the fact that I was overweight. When people used to say, "Jim Garlow is a 'heavy' preacher," they weren't just talking about the content of my sermons! In spite of my recent experience, I don't consider myself an expert in the area of weight loss. But I have learned this important lesson: there is an unmistakable connection between body and spirit. Our physical health and our spiritual well being are intimately connected. I have learned, too, the choices that we make in our habits, diet, and patterns of exercise have a tremendous effect upon our health *and* our ability to experience divine healing. The Apostle Paul described our bodies as a temple of the Holy Spirit, but at eighty pounds overweight, my "temple" was much bigger than the Holy Spirit needed! Because our bodies truly are the temple of the Holy Spirit, the way that we treat our bodies has serious implications for our physical and spiritual health. Our lifestyle can significantly affect our ability to experience God's healing power.

FAITH VERSUS PRESUMPTION

For years I was overweight, and I experienced some minor health problems as a result. During that time I found it difficult to speak authoritatively on the subjects of health in general and weight loss in particular. The reason is simple: I knew that I was not doing what I should have been in that area of my life. My habits of diet and exercise were not conducive to good health. Health problems from arthritis to diabetes to heart disease are affected by our lifestyle, particularly our weight. Other serious health problems result from unhealthy choices such as overeating, using tobacco or alcohol, or abusing drugs. People sometimes wonder if God heals us from these diseases, which are often directly related to our own poor choices and behaviors.

To consider that question, let's look at the difference between *faith* and *presumption*. Faith is the confidence that God will do what he has said he will do. Faith is the attitude that believes God still heals and that his healing power is available to us today. God has said that he does heal, and faith believes that he will. You might say that faith is holding God to what he has said he will do.

> It is presumptuous to demand God's healing when we continue to make unhealthy choices.

Presumption, on the other hand, holds God to what we want him to do. When Jesus was tempted in the wilderness, Satan took him to the highest point on the temple and told him to throw himself down, believing that God would catch him. Satan said, "For it is written: 'He will command his angels concerning you to guard you carefully . . . so that you will not strike your foot against a stone'" (Luke 4:9–10). The scripture was correctly cited but wrongly applied. Thus Jesus realized that it would be presumptuous to expect God to do that, since that was not really what was intended. Jesus replied, "Do not put the Lord your God to the test" (Luke 4:12).

In the same way, we are presumptuous when we claim God's promise of healing in the face of our own repeated poor choices or unhealthy lifestyles. It is true that God can cure any ailment including heart disease or cancer. Yet it is presumptuous to live an unhealthy lifestyle, ignoring God's command to honor him with our bodies, and then expect that he will miraculously provide good health. It makes no sense to abuse our bodies and then pray for a miracle. To place ourselves in a position to receive God's healing power, we are responsible to exercise good judgment. That applies particularly to obesity but also to other lifestyle-related illnesses. When we honor God with our bodies, it is not presumptuous to claim his healing power over disease.

ENHANCING HEALING

Through my recent experience of weight loss, I've discovered some lifestyle choices that significantly affect health. As with all of the principles related in this book, they are not laws. Practicing these behaviors is not a guarantee of good health, but living according to these precepts will improve the likelihood of experiencing health.

RESOLVE

After years of failure at maintaining proper weight, I was finally able to succeed. That victory came, frankly, from desperation. One day I said to myself, "I am not going to live like this the rest of my life."

Several years ago when the Billy Graham team came to San Diego to prepare for the Billy Graham Crusade, the organizers were amazed that in just four months the pastors and the Christians leaders of this community could prepare for the crusade. They said, "How is this possible? It generally takes so much longer." I answered, "It's because we're desperate for a spiritual awakening." When you are truly desperate—tired of living an unhealthy lifestyle—you will be spiritually ready to make the changes that promote good health.

Accountability

In order to succeed at weight loss, I had to acknowledge my need for help. Many years ago I had lost some weight. I thought I could do it again, but I couldn't. I needed other people to help me. I joined a weight-loss group and humbly admitted to myself that I couldn't do it alone. We need each other. That's the way God made us. When you join yourself with others who support you and keep you accountable, you'll be much more likely to succeed in establishing a healthy lifestyle.

Skill

The first lesson I learned in my weight-loss class was that willpower is ineffective in producing results. Our leader stood before us and said, "You don't have to have willpower to succeed. If you had willpower, you wouldn't be here in the first place. What you need is *skill* power." By carefully following the advice of my instructors and physician, I was able to lose eighty pounds in twenty-two weeks. When you admit that you don't know all that you need to know, you place yourself in a position to learn. And when you learn how to live in a healthier manner, using your God-given freedom to make wiser choices, you will succeed.

Fellowship

We all need encouragement. In my weight-loss program, I thrived on the encouragement of fellow class members. For the spiritual support that you need to experience health and healing, it is essential that you become part of a local church, worshiping regularly with other believers and gaining support and encouragement from them. If you do not attend church, you are missing a significant source of support for living a healthy lifestyle.

VISION

During the difficult times, I was motivated to continue losing weight by a powerful vision. I kept in my closet a suit that I had purchased when I was a graduate student almost three decades ago. I had purchased the suit in London, and it had a European cut. It was a very sleek suit. And I had a dream that I could wear that suit again. More than fitting into the suit, I wanted to become more healthy. What a blessing that will be to my family, I thought. That dream kept me motivated. Finally the day came, and I wore the suit again. That was thrilling for me, yet I have remained cautious. I have also kept one of my larger suits to remind me that if I become careless, I will have to wear it again.

Envision yourself in better health. See yourself thirty pounds lighter. Imagine your life without dependence upon tobacco or alcohol. Get God's vision of the future, and keep pursuing it.

HEALTHY THOUGHTS

Perhaps the most significant thing you can do to support healthy changes in your lifestyle is to change the way you think. Wrong thinking produces wrong results. Understanding right principles produces right results. When we think—that is, believe—the wrong things, we fail. But what if we were to think like "losers"—meaning think like people who really do *lose* weight? What if we make mental changes to support our physical desires? The results of doing just that were dramatic in my life, and they will be in yours as well. Here are some of the healthy thoughts that support a healthy lifestyle. Some of these statements are original, and some I've borrowed from other teachers. Focus on these key words to support your lifestyle changes.

When we choose a healthy lifestyle, we place ourselves in a position to receive healing.

- *Thinking*—If I change my mind, I will change my behavior. Ultimately, the fat is in my head.

- *Desperation*—My capacity to change is in direct proportion to the desperation I feel. Am I truly tired of living this way?

- *Passion*—Passion is my fuel; it empowers my action.

- *Strategy*—Strategy is my guide; it directs my passion toward a goal.

- *Acknowledge*—Three words will change my life: "I need help."

- *Humility*—It's not about me.

- *Vision*—I am able to see what I can become.

- *Ownership*—I didn't create my body, and it doesn't belong to me. I am a steward of it; therefore, I will treat it accordingly.

- *Excuses*—I can have excuses or I can have results, but I cannot have both.

- *Results*—I chose to make decisions that yield results.

- *Decisions*—I will pay attention to even small, seemingly inconsequential decisions because they have a cumulative effect.

- *Change*—I can change; I do not have to remain as I am.

- *Skill*—Due to my lack of will power, I will need to develop "skill power."

- *Records*—Keeping accurate daily records is a way of saying I value life.

- *Parameters*—Since I did not build adequate fences around my habits in the past, well established parameters are my friends in the present.

- *Exercise*—I do not like exercise, but I love *having* exercised. Therefore, I choose to be an active person.

- *Pleasure*—I can have either pleasure now and pain later, or discipline now and pleasure later.

- *Discipline*—Discipline gives me the dreams of my heart. Lack of discipline is a dream destroyer.

- *Consequences*—Bad actions yield bad consequences. Good actions yield good consequences. I choose good consequences, thus I choose good actions.

- *Momentum*—Momentum is a friend that I will cherish and protect.

- *Learning*—I choose to learn daily.

- *Silence*—I am not the teacher. I am the student. I will ask questions or remain silent.

- *Opinion*—This year, my goal is to have 20 percent fewer opinions.

- *Favorites*—I will limit myself to enjoy only those things that do not detract from my goals.

- *Routine*—In order to break free from a destructive rut, I will establish new health routines.

- *Variety*—I will be sufficiently creative to discover variety within the parameters set for me.

- *Success*—I will not allow my successes to set me up for failure.

- *Failure*—I will not allow my failures to make me think I cannot succeed.

- *Affirmation*—I accept the affirmations of others that encourage healthy habits.

- *Compliments*—While I appreciate compliments, I choose to live by eternal principles rather than the opinions of others concerning me.

- *Fear*—Although I chose to avoid unhealthy fears, I embrace the healthy fear that will restrain me from doing things that harm myself.

- *Criticism*—When I am doing what is right and healthy for me, I will not react to or be deterred by the criticism of others.

- *Endurance*—I can outlast the problem I am overcoming.

- *Preferences*—Preferences can be my friend, but I will not allow them to be my master.

- *Convictions*—Preferences are something I live by; convictions are what I will die for.

- *Principles*—Principles are to me what tracks are to a train: they guide me toward my goal.

- *Hope*—Hope holds me steady through difficult times.

- *Hunger*— I refuse to allow bodily hunger to rule my life.

- *Mind*—My mind rules over my body.

- *Spirit*—My spirit rules over my mind, which rules over my body.

- *Focus*—I choose to fill my mind with wholesome thoughts that produce healthy results.

- *Meditation*—My spirit was created for thinking higher thoughts.

- *Ongoing*—I accept the fact that I must always keep on keeping on.

Finding Healing

I am embarrassed to admit that I did not exercise regularly for twenty years. Now I exercise daily. For years I ate many sweets. Now I eat large quantities of fruits and vegetables. I'm healthier now than I was two years ago. With God's help, I will be even healthier two years from now. I know that the decisions I have made in the past were a detriment to my physical, emotional, and spiritual health. And I realize that the healthier choices I am now making have brought me to a better, more satisfying place in life. I thank God that he is faithful to me even when I behave selfishly and make poor choices, yet I am not presumptuous to believe that I can flout God's principles for living and always expect him to perform a miracle. I have discovered that when I live according to God's Word and do my best to honor him with my body, I place myself in a position to experience his healing power. But I don't want to always be in need of healing. I want to walk in health.

The same can be true for you.

LET'S PRAY

Father—

I resolve to make my body the temple of your Holy Spirit. I rejoice that you are willing to live within me, and I desire to honor you with my body. Give me wisdom to make wise choices, and surround me with friends who will hold me accountable. Forgive my failures in this area of my life, and enable me to do what I can to preserve the life and health that you have given.

In Jesus' name I ask this.

Amen.

For small group discussion questions on this chapter and additional resources on healing, visit www.wesleyan.org/gsh.

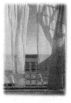

NINETEEN

ARE DEMONS REAL?

*Demons are real and cause chaos and
disorder, including illness.*

---

*Tammy and Ella had been friends since they were both
toddlers in the church nursery. Now high school seniors,
Tammy sensed that her friend had been drifting away from
God—and from her.*

*A couple of weeks earlier, Ella had tried to convince
Tammy to go to a party where there would be fortune telling,
but Tammy didn't feel right about it. "I have homework," she
said. "Besides, that's stuff is kinda freaky."*

One day Ella didn't show up for school. That afternoon, Tammy called Ella's house. Her mother answered.

"This is Tammy. Is Ella OK? I noticed she wasn't at school today."

"Thanks for calling, Tammy. Actually, Ella is sick, but we're not sure what's wrong. She's just been acting a little strange. I'm sure she'd like a visitor."

The moment Tammy entered Ella's bedroom, she could tell something was wrong with her friend. More than that, she sensed a strange presence in the room—something evil.

"Ella . . . are you all right?"

"Get away from me," Ella hissed. "Get out!"

Tammy backed slowly toward the door. "This isn't like Ella," she thought. "What in the world is going on here?"

This is a book about healing; it is not a book about deliverance. Yet deliverance often times precedes healing. Thus we need to know something about deliverance in order to understand divine healing. At the risk of being misunderstood, I will reduce to a few pages a discussion of this topic, which merits an extended treatment.

A word of caution is appropriate at this point. There are two extremes, two "ditches," that we must avoid falling into. First, we should not be quick to assume that an ill person suffers from demonic affliction. It is an error to see demons as the cause of every malady. That is harmful because it may divert attention from the true cause. Those who fall into this ditch look for a demon under every rock. They obsess with the thought that "Satan is attacking me." We need to stay out of that ditch.

On the other side of the road is the ditch of denial. This is an unwillingness to admit either that demons exist or that they might be involved in our world or that a demon could oppress a Christian. Those who fall into this error dismiss major passage of the New Testament. Both obsession with demons and denial of them are errors. Let's avoid both.

ABOUT DEMONS

What are demons? We don't know for certain. Some contend they are fallen angels. Others see them simply as disembodied spirits. They do appear to be organized by some ranking or hierarchical structure in the spirit realm. Some contend that the existence of demons is merely the construct of a primitive and superstitious world. They insist that demons do not exist and that no sophisticated mind would believe that they did. Some go so far as to say that Jesus only pretended to believe that demons were real because he was dealing with unsophisticated people. According to this theory, Jesus knew that people who were "delivered" were really suffering from psychological problems.

I believe that Jesus did, in fact, accept the existence of a demonic realm and that he understood that realm to be populated by Satan and his demonic hordes. Jesus felt it was important to teach his followers how to deliver people from demon activity. Distasteful as the subject may be, we, too, should learn how to pray for people so they may be delivered.

There is a spiritual world that we cannot see, and that world includes dark spiritual forces.

DEMONS AND THE NEW TESTAMENT

The New Testament uses several phrases to describe a person who is affected by demon. People are variously described as demonized, having unclean spirits, having demons, being troubled by unclean spirits, afflicted, seized by a spirit, being entered by demons, being entered by Satan, and even being filled by Satan.

Can a believer be troubled by demons? Most people would say, "No." We usually reason that if a person is filled with Christ, he or she cannot be possessed by a demon at the same time. Yet we arrive at the wrong conclusion because we frame the question incorrectly.

> Jesus Christ has already won the battle over Satan and his forces.

As I have stated often, my mentor in learning about these issues was John Wimber. Wimber asserted that demon activity rarely results in demon *possession*. That is why I prefer never to use the term *possession*. I prefer the term *demon affliction* instead. What is the difference? This term allows us to see demonization on a continuum with varying degrees rather than an all-or-nothing condition.

Consider this analogy. After consuming a small amount of alcohol, a person experiences some physical effects such as relaxation. After consuming more alcohol, motor skills are affected. Speech may become slurred. Reactions are slowed. Finally, after consuming a large amount of alcohol, a person may lose consciousness. So the term *alcohol impaired* may be more useful for describing the effects of alcohol than is the term *drunk*.

Demonic affliction is similar in that it can exist in varying degrees. It may result in only minor evidences if a demon is harassing a person. Or it may result in dramatic symptoms if a person is truly "possessed" by a demon.

ENTRY POINTS

How do demons gain access to a person's life? Frankly, we don't always know, but here is a partial list of some of some ways in which demon affliction can begin.

Carnal Desires. Often indulged to excess, things like lust, stealing, lying, and gluttony can be areas in which Satan gains a foothold in a person's life.

Individual Vulnerabilities. Each of us has chinks in our spiritual armor, vulnerable areas in our emotional or psychological lives caused by unusual trauma. This vulnerabilities may break down our normal, healthy spiritual defenses.

Involvement in the Occult. Delving into witchcraft or the occult opens the door for demon involvement in our lives.

Alcohol or Drug Abuse. The abuse of alcohol or drugs can lead to addiction, a clear entry point for demonic activity.

Sexual Promiscuity. Whether done *by* us or done *to* us, sexual sin has powerful consequences in the lives of all concerned and can be a point of entry for demonic activity.

ABOUT DELIVERANCE

When should we pray for someone to be delivered from demon affliction? Here are some indications. First, when someone is involved in compulsive behavior and cannot stop. Also when a person simply knows that he or she has a demon. Another clue to demon affliction is bizarre behavior. A more obvious indicator—but one that occurs *infrequently*—is when a demon manifests itself by speaking through a person's vocal cords. Those most seasoned in deliverance know that in those rare cases where that occurs, the one leading the deliverance needs to first silence the demon, insisting that the demon not speak.

However, before assuming that deliverance is needed, make certain that the person who appears to be afflicted is practicing basic Christian disciplines such as prayer, Bible reading, fasting, receiving the Eucharist, participation in fellowship or accountability groups, tithing, ministry, and witnessing. Some people mistakenly assume they "have a demon" when the real reason for their spiritual failure is lack of discipline.

PRESERVING DIGNITY AND PRIVACY

Tragically deliverance has sometimes been trivialized, made fun of, or exploited. We should take the notion of demonic affliction seriously without yielding to the temptation to grandstand our success in this area. Also, it is important never to place blame on the person needing deliverance. We should respect that person's dignity and privacy. Deliverance should not be done in a public setting unless conditions dictate.

Deliverance does not consist of yelling, panting, or weird chanting as seen in some popular movies. These images of deliverance have caused many Christians to be so afraid of deliverance that they do not follow the practice established by Jesus and his earliest followers.

PRAYING FOR DELIVERANCE

In order to be delivered from demon affliction, the person must want to be delivered. Those involved in demonic deliverance have discovered an unusual phenomenon: it helps if the demon's name (which is usually a tendency or action, such as the "demon of alcohol" or "demon of lust") is known.

Deliverance begins with earnest prayer and fasting. It is best to pray as a team, not alone. Pray for protection over all involved. Gently, lovingly lead the person needing deliverance in prayer for any unconfessed sins that may exist in his or her life. Attempt to see if there is unforgiveness, bitterness, or resentment that might be serving as a type of fortress behind which the Enemy is allowed to hide.

Use straightforward and simple language, such as "I command this evil spirit to come out in the Name of Jesus. I command, by God's authority, for this spirit to depart without harming this person or any others and without creating a disturbance. And I send this spirit to Jesus Christ that he might dispose of it as he will." It is not necessary to yell. The key is the power of Christ—nothing more, nothing less. We have no authority. Jesus has all authority. The authority we exercise is that which he has graciously given to us. When we talk to God, we ask. When we talk to demons, we command. Do not confuse the two methods. We never have the right to command God. But God does give us authority over demons.

SUCCESSFUL DELIVERANCE

How will we know if we have been successful? The demon-afflicted person will know—either immediately or days later. Do not claim deliverance. Let time indicate whether or not the demonic spirit was successfully removed. And do not become discouraged if the attempt at deliverance is not successful. Continue praying, believing, and—if God directs—fasting.

AFTER DELIVERANCE

When a person has been set free from demonic affliction, pray that her or she will be filled with the wonderful Spirit of the Living God. Instruct the person how to walk in freedom. Strongly encourage him or her to practice the standard Christian disciplines mentioned above.

FINAL ADVICE

Here is a final and critically important admonition: Do not become enamored with deliverance. That was the warning given by Jesus to the seventy disciples who returned from a successful mission trip. They were amazed at their newfound power over demons, and Jesus told them, "Do not rejoice that the spirits submit to you, but rejoice that your names are written in heaven" (Luke 10:20). It is true that Jesus gives us the authority to pray for the deliverance of those who are demon afflicted. But don't gloat about that power. Instead, delight in the one who gives that power.

LET'S PRAY

Father—

Your Word has promised that the power of darkness will not stand in the presence of Jesus. In Christ, I claim protection from the Enemy. I praise you, Most High God, for your might and power and strength. And I thank you for the love that surrounds me and all who believe in you. Deliver us from evil, I pray, in Jesus' name.

Amen.

For small group discussion questions on this chapter and additional resources on healing, visit www.wesleyan.org/gsh.

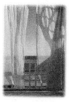

CAN SICKNESS HAVE A SPIRITUAL CONNECTION FROM ONE GENERATION TO ANOTHER?

*The actions of any person can affect
generations to come.*

Everyone told Claudia Carson that turning thirty wasn't
so bad, but a week after her birthday she was starting to feel
old. First she felt lightheaded, then came the dizzy spells.

After another week, Claudia's mother stopped by for a
visit. "How are you, honey?" Norma Carson asked lightly.
"Is thirty as bad as you thought?"

"Actually, it's worse. I keep getting dizzy. I don't know
what's wrong with me."

Norma's expression became serious. "Dizzy spells?"

"Yeah, I've had them for almost two weeks," Claudia said. "Maybe I should go to a doctor."

"Yes," Norma said, "you should. Maybe he can help you more than he did me?"

"Mom, what are you talking about?"

"I had them too, honey. And so did your grandmother. I was hoping this . . . curse would skip a generation."

Claudia looked skeptical. "Come on, Mom. A family curse? You can't be serious."

How many times have you had younger people say something like "I will *never* be like my dad," or, "I can't stand that trait in my mother, and I'll never behave that way"? Most of the time, those same young people grow into adults that very much resemble their parents. We often grow up to become like our parents in ways that have nothing to do with hereditary issues, like height and hair color.

Why is that?

The reason is because of *familial spirits,* spirits that follow family lines (not to be confused with *familiar* spirits). Familial (from the word *family*) spirits can be a significant blockage to God's healing in our lives. When they are removed, it opens the channel for God's grace to flow to us. This concept is foreign to modern thinking, but it is founded in Scripture. Let's see what the Bible has to say about familial spirits and their connection to illness and healing.

CORPORATE RESPONSIBILITY

Individual actions can have corporate, or social, consequences. In some cases, the effects of one person's behavior can affect other people for generations to come. Two Scriptures in particular make that point.

Exodus 34:6–7 says, "And [the LORD] passed in front of Moses, proclaiming, 'The LORD, the LORD, the compassionate and gracious God, slow to anger, abounding in love and faithfulness, maintaining love to thousands, and forgiving wickedness, rebellion and sin. Yet he does not leave the guilty unpunished; he punishes the children and their children for the sin of the fathers to the third and fourth generation.'"

> Modern people dislike the notion of generational curses, yet the Bible speaks of them.

Numbers 14:18 says, "The LORD is slow to anger, abounding in love and forgiving sin and rebellion. Yet He does not leave the guilty unpunished; he punishes the children for the sin of the fathers to the third and fourth generation."

Those Scriptures don't sit well with most people in the modern world. Aren't we all supposed to be responsible for ourselves? It seems unfair that someone could be punished or suffer for the actions of another. That thinking goes against what we have been taught about freedom and responsibility. We are individualistic in our thinking. "What I do is nobody's business but my own," we often think.

But what you do does make a difference to others. In the Bible, sin is often seen as a corporate (or social) act, regardless of whether it was committed by one person or many. The actions of one person could have a great impact on others; there was no such thing as a private sin.

That is true today. If the president of a nation lies, the spirit of deception is released across the land. Other leaders will be less honest, and children will lie more. If a pastor commits adultery, that act may affect a congregation for years to come. People who are not yet born may feel the impact of that sin. Principals, parents, teachers, brothers, and sisters can affect many people with their wrongdoing.

All sin is "societal" in that it has an impact on others. There is no such thing as "private" sin.

How does that apply to healing? Think, for example, of the tremendous impact of sexual sin upon a family. You may know of cases in which the children, grandchildren, and even great grandchildren of a man or woman were impacted by sins such as rape, incest, or child abuse. The effects of that sin can be manifested in emotional distress, mental illness, and even physical illness for generations. The things we do affect other people. Therefore, we may suffer the effects of sin committed by those who came before us.

CORPORATE BLESSING

The transgenerational impact of sin causes some to wonder about the character of God. "What kind of God would punish children for the sins of their ancestors?" they ask. The answer is that he is a God of love and compassion, for he also wants to pour out blessings from generation to generation. When the effects of transgenerational sin are removed, God's blessings can be released, including the blessing of healing.

Deuteronomy 7:9 says, "Know therefore that the LORD your God is God; he is the faithful God, keeping his covenant of love to a thousand generations of those who love him and keep his commands." When the Bible describes God's judgment upon sin, it talks about three and four generations.

> God desires to bless you, your children, and your children's children.

Yet when the Bible describes God's blessings, it mentions a thousand generations. That would be about thirty thousand years. That's a nice way of saying that God's blessings simply have no end.

God's love for you is intense. His passion for you has no ending point. He does not desire that a "family-line spirit" should afflict you and your family for years to come. What he wants is to bless you.

We see that illustrated in the book of Isaiah. This prophet's message was one of judgment. Isaiah spoke to God's people at a time when they needed to hear some tough preaching. He told them that if they didn't obey God, their entire nation would be punished. That was corporate, or societal, responsibility. The first thirty-nine chapters of Isaiah contain a stern message.

However, in Isaiah 40, everything changes. The remainder of the book is a love song for God's people. Isaiah describes the wonderful blessings that God has in store for them. The second half of the book opens with these tender words, "Comfort, comfort my people, says your God. Speak tenderly to Jerusalem, and proclaim to her that her hard service has been completed, that her sin has been paid for, that she has received from the LORD's hand double for all her sins" (Isa. 40:1–2). In other words, be tender with God's people. The debt is paid. It is time to receive God's blessings. That's the nature of our God, and he loves to see us set free and the power of familial spirits broken.

FINDING FREEDOM

As mentioned in chapter 3, I once prayed for a pastor who suffered from a ringing in his ears. The problem was so intense that when he stood behind the pulpit to preach, he was almost unable to hear his own words. He wanted healing. "What more can you tell me about this?" I asked.

"All I know," he answered, "is that my brothers all have it, and my father had it as well." That was very likely the result of a familial spirit—an affliction that was passed from one generation to the next. Remember that before dealing with the physical, it is necessary to deal with the spiritual. In this case, the man had to be set free from the sin of the past before he could be healed from his present ailment.

When dealing with a familial spirit, ask the Lord to reveal the problem so that it can be dealt with. Pray, "Lord, please show us if the

Enemy made some kind of foothold in this family. Reveal it to us so that we can rebuke that in the name of Jesus and see this person set free." When you break the power of the past in Jesus' name, God's healing can be released in the present, and healing can come. We do not need to labor under the curse of a familial spirit. As children of God's New Covenant, we can claim our freedom in Jesus' name.

LET'S PRAY

Father—

I have sinned against you, and not I alone. My parents, and their parents, and their parents before them were willful and disobedient. I pray that you would forgive our sins and release your blessing upon us—life, and health, and peace.

In Jesus' name I ask this.

Amen.

For small group discussion questions on this chapter and additional resources on healing, visit www.wesleyan.org/gsh.

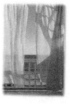

HOW LONG
SHOULD I
WAIT TO BE HEALED?

Lack of persistence in prayer is a significant reason
some people are not healed.

"*I guess people hold on to hope any way they can,*"
Charlie mused as he read the prayer requests in the church
bulletin. He and Margaret had been attending Faith
Community Church for five years, and every Sunday there
was a prayer request for Tyler Carson.

Tyler had been born with normal vision but had lost
his sight over several years. Now seven years old, he was
completely blind. "*We know God will heal him,*" Tyler's

mother would say. "We just don't know when."

Charlie shook his head sadly. "After five years," he thought, "it's time to accept reality."

During the prayer-and-praise time, Tyler's mom went to the microphone. "Pastor, I just want to thank everybody for their faithful prayer." She paused, trying to keep her composure. "We went to the doctor this week . . . and Tyler could see light—and some shapes. God is doing a miracle in our little boy."

The congregation burst into applause. "Well I'll be," Charlie said. "I never would have believed it."

What do you do when someone is not healed for a long time? It can be discouraging to do your best to walk with the Father, pray diligently for healing, and yet see a loved one continue to suffer and become sicker. How long should we pray for healing? Is there a point where we should simply give up and say, "It's not going to happen this time"?

Tommy Tyson, a Methodist evangelist, has coined the term *soaking prayer*. By that, he means praying persistently and saturating the issue with fervent prayer. Galatians 6:9 says, "Let us not become weary in doing good, for at the proper time we will reap a harvest if we do not give up." And Hebrews 10:36 says, "You need to persevere so that when you have done the will of God, you will receive what he has promised." One reason why some people are not healed is that we lack importunity in prayer. We do not pray persistently or with enough patience. We give up too easily and, as a result, do not see the release of God's healing power. A key to praying effectively for healing is to pray persistently.

The Need for Importunity

Daniel 10:12–13 records this amazing event: "Then he said to me, 'Do not be afraid, Daniel. Since the first day that you set your mind to gain understanding and to humble yourself before your God, your words were heard, and I have come in response to them. But the prince of the Persian kingdom resisted me twenty-one days. Then Michael, one of the chief princes, came to help me, because I was detained there with the king of Persia." For twenty-one days, Daniel prayed and got no response. The reason is that there was a battle taking place in the spiritual world that Daniel knew nothing about.

That is often the case in our prayers for healing. We see only half of the equation. We see the physical world. It is true that God sometimes reveals to us what he is doing; we always try to discern where God is at work and join him there. Yet we do not see all that happens in the spiritual world. In Daniel's case the delay lasted twenty-one days. Could it be longer in some cases? A year? Five years? Twenty years? Indeed it could. That is why we need to be persistent in prayer, even when we see no immediate results.

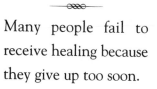

Many people fail to receive healing because they give up too soon.

I do not know the reason, but most healing today is not accomplished instantly. As discussed in a preceding chapter, most healing comes gradually. Instantaneous miracles do occur, but not often. That's puzzling because in the New Testament, the situation seems to be reversed. Most miracles happened immediately. Only a few took place gradually. So in our day, there is a greater need for persistence in prayer. We must pray and not give up. As mentioned previously, I struggled for years with a respiratory ailment. Many people prayed for my healing. It finally came, but after thirteen long years.

THE CALL OF SCRIPTURE

Several Scripture passages make a direct appeal for us to be importunate—that is, to be assertive and persistent in our prayers. Let's examine a few, beginning with Luke 11:5–10.

> Then he said to them, "Suppose one of you has a friend, and he goes to him at midnight and says, 'Friend, lend me three loaves of bread, because a friend of mine on a journey has come to me, and I have nothing to set before him.'
>
> "Then the one inside answers, 'Don't bother me. The door is already locked, and my children are with me in bed. I can't get up and give you anything.' I tell you, though he will not get up and give him the bread because he is his friend, yet because of the man's boldness he will get up and give him as much as he needs.
>
> "So I say to you: Ask and it will be given to you; seek and you will find; knock and the door will be opened to you. For everyone who asks receives; he who seeks finds; and to him who knocks, the door will be opened."

Some translations say that it is because of the visitor's *persistence* that he will receive as much as he needs. This is placed in Luke's gospel right after the teaching on the Lord's Prayer. So in Luke's mind, there is a strong tie between prayer and persistence.

Let's look at another example. Luke 18:1–8 relates a similar teaching:

> Then Jesus told his disciples a parable to show them that they should always pray and not give up. He said: "In a certain town there was a judge who neither feared God nor cared

about men. And there was a widow in that town who kept coming to him with the plea, 'Grant me justice against my adversary.'

For some time he refused. But finally he said to himself, 'Even though I don't fear God or care about men, yet because this widow keeps bothering me, I will see that she gets justice, so that she won't eventually wear me out with her coming!'"

And the Lord said, "Listen to what the unjust judge says. And will not God bring about justice for his chosen ones, who cry out to him day and night? Will he keep putting them off? I tell you, he will see that they get justice, and quickly."

Being persistent in prayer is not the same as begging God in the way a child begs a parent: "Please, please, please give me what I want!" Remember that God really does love us and wants us to be well. There are a number of potential blockages to healing, so when we are not healed immediately, it does not mean that God wants us sick. By being persistent in prayer, we demonstrate our faith in God. We call out to him as a child to a loving parent, believing that he really does want to release his healing power to us. When we pray and don't give up, we show ourselves to have faith.

Isn't that what we would do in any other area? When we pray for the salvation of a loved one, we don't give up just because there is no response in a week, month, or even a few years? We pray diligently for that person, believing that God wants his or her salvation even more than we do. The challenge for us in praying for healing is to be persistent. We must not become discouraged or doubt God's goodness when some are not healed. We need to continue to pray.

DON'T GIVE UP

To encourage you to keep praying for healing, I will relate a very personal story. As I have stated, one of the people who has most affected my thinking on the subject of divine healing is John Wimber, the late founder of the Vineyard Fellowship. As mentioned in the preface, during the 1980s, Wimber taught at Fuller Theological Seminary and began to see an explosion of the Holy Spirit's work in the area of healing. He was teaching a class entitled "Signs and Wonders and Church Growth."

> When you pray, ask for God's healing—then ask again, and again, and again.

During the class, John said, "We've been talking about healing, so why don't we pray for the sick." People got well that day. So the next class day, they did the same thing, and people got well again. The word spread, and soon people were attending the class who weren't enrolled. The crowd became so large that they had to limit attendance. Some time later I took the course. It had been moved to a new venue, and some three thousand of us attended. We saw amazing signs and wonders, including healing. John Wimber began to travel and teach people to pray for the sick, and he influenced many people—including me.

Another person influenced by the teaching of John Wimber was an Anglican priest from England named David Watson. Watson and Wimber traveled throughout England and saw thousands healed. Then David Watson became ill with cancer. John and others prayed for him, but he became more ill. Finally, John Wimber said to his friend, "David, you're about to die."

David said, "Yes."

John asked, "David, what am I going to tell the people about healing?"

And among David Watson's last words were these: "Tell the people to keep praying for the sick."

A number of years ago, my wife and I attended the funeral for John Wimber. Although I seldom become emotional, I was so grieved by the loss of this man who had taught me so much that I cried throughout the entire service. I kept thinking to myself, "I wonder what John would say, or what did he say, about the health problems he suffered that finally took his life. The only words that came to my mind were these, the last words of David Watson: "Keep praying for the sick."

It doesn't add up in our minds. In most cases we have no clear explanation for why one person is healed and another isn't, or why some people must suffer for years before they experience healing. We face disappointments in this area, and we wonder.

Yet we must keep on praying for the sick. We know that God is a loving Father. We know that he desires to bless us. We seek him with all of our heart. And we leave to him the mystery of spiritual healing. We pray for those who are ill—and we don't give up.

At the risk of being misunderstood or ridiculed, I will share the fact that I have been praying for the miraculous healing of my nephew, now twenty-two years old, who is afflicted with Down's syndrome. Has he been healed? No. Will he be healed? I do not know. Yet I will continue to pray for him until one of us is placed in the arms of God.

Let's Pray

Father—

It has been such a long, long time—and still we are waiting. We long for health and wholeness. We ask for relief from pain. We wish for energy and strength to be renewed in us.

We believe, Lord, that you have the power to heal, and we ask you again: Release your healing power upon those who are in need. Release your healing power upon me. Make me whole.

In Jesus' name I ask this.

Amen.

For small group discussion questions on this chapter and additional resources on healing, visit www.wesleyan.org/gsh.

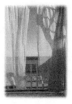

PART FOUR

How to Pray
For the Sick

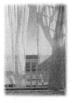

WHERE DO I BEGIN?

*Holy Spirit–saturated worship creates
the atmosphere for healing.*

"*I better sit out the next session,*" *Carol said, sitting
across the lunch table from her husband.* "*I feel a headache
coming on.*" *She closed her eyes, rubbing her temples.*

*Jim and Carol were in Anaheim for a weeklong
conference on worship. For three days they had studied
the Word, worshiped with other believers almost
constantly, and enjoyed the presence of the Holy Spirit
like never before.*

But by the middle of the third day, Carol's temples were throbbing. "I hate to miss what's happening," she lamented, "but I just don't feel well."

Without a word, Jim placed a hand on his wife's forehead. "In the name of Jesus, headache, be gone!" he pronounced.

Carol blinked. "That's amazing," she said. "What did you just do? The pain is gone."

"I didn't do anything," Jim said calmly. "We've been in the presence of the Holy Spirit for three days. That takes care of a lot of problems."

It is I, Carol, who is described in that story. I was instantly healed of that headache when Jim prayed a prayer of pronouncement on my behalf. While a headache may seem like a small thing, believe me, it was not. I felt very ill, but God healed me in a moment. Yet I am convinced that my healing was not truly instantaneous in one sense. It followed days of Scripture study, prayer, teaching, and worship. We were spiritually cleansed and drawn closer to God. Being in a Spirit-saturated environment set the stage for what seemed like an immediate release of God's healing power.

That event changed my perspective on healing prayer. Like most Christians, I have longed to see instant answers to prayer for healing—miracles on demand. I have learned that most healing comes gradually. But more important, I have learned that seeking God through worship is a critically important component of healing prayer. When we are united with the Father in worship, we are far more likely to see healing occur.

After making that discovery, I decided to apply the principle in a class I was teaching at our church. Rather than majoring the session on teaching, we would devote most of our time to worship, starting with Scripture reading. At the beginning of the class, I explained the format for the evening, then asked members to listen as I read Isaiah 45. I simply read the text with soft instrumental music playing in the background. I continued by reading John 15:9–13 and two stories of Jesus healing the sick from Luke 5. Then we sang together. The remainder of the class was spent in prayer.

Attending the class that evening was a woman whose cancer had been declared terminal, a man just diagnosed with neuropathy, and two women dealing with emotional trauma. We formed small groups around the room to petition the Lord for these and other individual concerns. We didn't see any instantaneous miracles. Yet all members of the class sensed that God was present. We had experienced deep communion with the Holy God through Scripture reading, worship, and prayer. We had confidence that our prayers had been heard and that God would answer. Worship became our gateway to effective prayer.

We would all like to see instantaneous healing. That's always our desire. But for some reason, God prefers to take us through a process of character building first. He begins with our inner healing, and then moves to healing of the body. The presence of the Holy Spirit is always necessary for healing to take place. Where the Holy Spirit is present, healing occurs. So worship is a vital component of prayer for healing. When we seek after God and enter into his presence, we place ourselves in a position to be healed.

Seeking God's Healing Power

Every day people pick up a phone or sit in front of a doctor to be given a bad report about their health. You may have heard those heart-rending words yourself and realized that you were facing an issue of life and death. How did you cope when you realized you were facing a problem for which you had no resources—for which even your physician was ill-equipped to solve? Your conversation with a doctor could not have answered all the questions you have about your body and what is happening to you. Perhaps you were left with a sense of fear and the overwhelming question, "What am I to do?"

It is normal to react initially with fear, despair, or hopelessness when facing an overwhelming situation. Often David begins his psalms with despairing cries like this one, "Save me, O God, for the waters have come up to my neck. I sink in the miry depths, where there is no foothold. I have come into the deep waters; the floods engulf me. I am worn out calling for help; my throat is parched. My eyes fail, looking for my God" (Ps. 69:1–3).

> If healing accompanies the Holy Spirit, then worship is the place to begin seeking healing.

Yet amid those desperate cries we find also the promises of God. "Blessed is he who has regard for the weak; the LORD delivers him in times of trouble. The LORD will protect him and preserve his life; he will bless him in the land and not surrender him to the desire of his foes. The LORD will sustain him on his sickbed and restore him from his bed of illness" (Ps. 41:1–3).

OPEN YOURSELF TO GOD'S POWER

God is a loving Father who desires to give good gifts to his children. His loving heart does hear and respond to your pleadings. His purpose for you does not include dwelling in sickness and hopelessness. Here is a picture of you and me when we face a situation that is far beyond our control:

> I see a big, blue sky with lots of fluffy, white clouds. A long arm is reaching through these clouds from the heavens toward me. I am frantically treading water amid the tumultuous waves of this huge ocean. My body is aching and tired.

I cannot go on any longer and am about to sink when a hand reaches for me and pulls me out of the deep waters (Psalm 18:9, 16 paraphrased).

God wants us to recognize the source of our comfort and to realize who it is that will go to battle for us. The pain and devastation of the diseases we face do not always immobilize us. Instead, it is fear and emotional pain that keep us from seeking help. It takes tremendous strength not to dwell in that place of fear. So when you feel the hand of God reaching for your hand, pulling you up, accept it, and you will immediately sense his presence washing over you.

Yet you must be open to God's healing power. If you are unwilling to open yourself to God's supernatural work in your life, you will not see his purpose accomplished in you. God desires a deep relationship with you. He wants you wholeheartedly. In this moment of need is a great opportunity for him to reveal more of himself to you.

CONSECRATE YOURSELF TO GOD

A clean heart, pure motives, and a spirit of repentance will allow God to freely perform awesome acts in your life. Sin can create a blockage for God's healing work in us. The book of Romans speaks of the connection of sin and death. Paul writes, "Don't you know that when you offer yourselves to someone to obey him as slaves, you are slaves to the one whom you obey—whether you are slaves to sin, which leads to death, or to obedience, which leads to righteousness?" (Rom. 6:16)

Thankfully, God's grace, mercy, and lovingkindness pave the way for us to be cleansed from our sin. For this to be accomplished, we must have a change of attitude in our inner spirit; our motives must be lined up with his, which are based upon his Word. When that happens, we can "hear joy and gladness," be restored to the joy of our salvation, and upheld by his generous Spirit (Ps. 51:8, 12).

Our goal is for God's hand to freely move in the hard places we face, providing hope and victory. When we consecrate ourselves to God, freely confessing our sin and dedicating our lives to him, we open ourselves to his healing power. Psalm 66:3, 4, 5, 10–12 says it best: "How awesome are your deeds! So great is your power that your enemies cringe before you. All the earth bows down to you; they sing praise to you, they sing praise to your name. Come and see what God has done, how awesome his works in man's behalf. . . . For you, O God, tested us; you refined us like silver. . . . We went through fire and water, but you brought us to a place of abundance."

SEEK GOD THROUGH WORSHIP

Worshiping God is the act that brings us into his presence. In the midst of a worship experience, you hear phrases like "Shout to the Lord all the earth, let us sing. Power and majesty, praise to the King." Or you may sing out words like "Great is the Lord, and great is his mercy." The words and music lift your spirits with exuberance that causes you to enter a higher level in your relationship with God. While meditating on the words of Isaiah 40:31—"Those who hope in the LORD will renew their strength. They will soar on wings like eagles; they will run and not grow weary, they will walk and not be faint"—you may sense God's strength flowing into you. You realize that you now have the strength to continue. Merely reading the first words of Psalm 23 can cause a soothing sense of comfort and well-being to wash over you.

Both of these mediums, Scripture and music, are acts of worship, and each can cause God's presence to descend from the heavens to the place where you are. Whatever style of music or translation of Scripture that ministers to you personally can become the conduit for God to reach out and touch you in your greatest need.

There may be times during the experience of worship when you recognize wrong attitudes toward others, unforgiveness, or sin in your heart that prevents you from fully giving yourself to God and acknowledging how wonderful he is. You may feel dead and lifeless. At that moment you can say to the Lord that you do not want anything blocking your adoration of him. Ask God's forgiveness, and then deal with each issue God brings to your attention. The worship of God is best expressed when repentance has cleansed the heart and purified the mind to enter the presence of God.

In receiving healing for myself and in ministering healing to others, I have discovered that a key component for the work of healing is clean, clear, direct access to God. Your desire for him and no other person or thing must be strong and compelling. Your worship says, "He is the Lord, and there is no other." For it is in this atmosphere of worship that the presence of God brings the power to heal. It does not come by any knowledge about healing or previous experience in praying for others. In fact, God seems to show himself in various forms and unique ways. We must be discerning and open to how God wants to bring healing to each individual.

Seek the Support of Others

After crying out to God in prayer over a difficult life issue, go to someone—a family member, friend, or fellow church member—for prayer support. It is thrilling to watch God's hand at work when these supporters come together in prayer at your home or church, or spend time in Scripture and prayer at a home group. Corporate healing services are spectacular opportunities to display unity and agreement with the body of Christ through Scripture study, worship, and prayer. While it is crucial for the individual dealing with the difficulty to dwell deeply in personal times of Scripture study, worship, and prayer with God, it is in the corporate setting that we gain love and support and feel great strength and power as our hearts are united as we lift up the name of Jesus.

The focus of prayer in these settings may likely not be on healing but on seeing what God wants to accomplish emotionally and spiritually in both those who pray and the one for whom they are praying. It may be that we are slow to grow spiritually, or simply that God takes his time in developing our character in order to accomplish his purpose for us. Either way, prayer takes time. To pray more effectively, we can only improve on our sensitivity to worship and listen to God's voice more carefully. Continually searching for Scripture verses that pertain to your particular life issue brings that Word of God into a positive, direct alignment with the solution God plans for your life.

A typical format for a prayer service for healing includes the study of a Scripture passage, followed by a time of worship, then prayer. Worshipers prepare themselves individually by spending quiet time alone in Scripture, worshiping and listening for God's Word. Sometimes fasting is needed before the prayer time. Those for whom prayer will be offered can also prepare their hearts and minds for prayer. They are encouraged to bring family and friends to support them. The constant objective is to allow God's presence and anointing to bring healing first to the soul and ultimately to the body.

Persevere

Our motto must be "Courage and perseverance keeps me moving forward." God honors and blesses those who set a course, learn how to handle their emotional and spiritual responses, and do not give up. Pain and suffering is part of the experience we will endure to find healing. Healing of the body does not always come in an instant. Trust in an almighty God must replace fear. Comfort and peace will banish anxiety and worry. Assurance that God's presence is with you will relieve despair. Whatever feeling is pulling you down, there is always a positive counterattack found in the Word of God.

To encourage and further release the victory of healing that is needed in your body, boldly declare the mighty work both spiritually and physically that God has done and continues to do in your life. Speaking Scripture aloud to others, especially skeptics, releases the power and might of God's Word over the negativity of Satan's devices. What a testimony to be able to praise the Lord in front of your family and friends, even strangers, of God's graciousness, mercy, and compassion over your devastation and despair!

DAN'S STORY

Dan, a man in his early thirties, often commented that he had led a boring Christian life. That changed when he was diagnosed with cancer. When tests revealed that Dan had cancer of the colon that may have spread to his liver, he was completely overwhelmed. "Satan began his attack on me," Dan said, "wanting me to fear dying and leaving my kids without a father. The only relief I received was praying to Jesus. After praying this way, I would often feel relief and be able to return to whatever it was I was doing."

> As we seek God, we move forward in spite of obstacles. Pray and don't give up.

A surgeon removed Dan's colon and performed a biopsy, which confirmed the diagnosis. Meanwhile, Dan's wife, Jenn, called for prayer from members of their family and church friends, organizing a prayer chain that included people in thirteen states, two countries, and about fifty churches. Hundreds of people were praying for Dan throughout his illness. Jenn and Dan sensed that they could trust God, and they believed in his healing power.

Then came more bad news. The cancer had spread to Dan's liver. "This was the major blow, and it hit me hard," Dan said. "But I still felt that God would take care of me. I told God that his job just got a whole lot bigger." Dan was determined to persevere.

Dan began chemotherapy, and his appearance went from trim and athletic to emaciated. He attended a healing service at his church, where the group experienced an extraordinary time of worship, bringing God's presence and healing power. The spirit of the Scripture pervaded the hearts and minds of those there, that the God of hope filled us with all joy and peace in believing that we could abound in hope by the power of the Holy Spirit (see Rom. 15:13). All who attended were inspired and changed. Shortly thereafter, an MRI showed amazing results. Dan's cancer had decreased rapidly in size. Four months later another MRI showed that Dan was cancer free.

Dan and Jenn report that they do not always understand why Dan was healed and others are not. Yet they know that their relationship with God has become deeper, and they are more than ever convinced of God's amazing power to heal. Dan's healing was not instantaneous, and it included medical treatments and surgery. Yet supported by prayer and empowered by worship, Dan knows that it was God's power that touched his body. They have seen the hand of God do its miraculous work and know that the Lord is great and greatly to be praised.

LET'S PRAY

Father—

I worship you in your splendor, power, holiness, and beauty. I surrender my life to you entirely. I lay all that I am and all that I have at your feet. I want you and you only. Fill me with your Holy Spirit, I pray.

In Jesus' name,

Amen.

For small group discussion questions on this chapter and additional resources on healing, visit www.wesleyan.org/gsh.

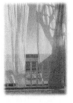

How Do
I Pray
For the Sick?

I must learn the steps to praying for healing.

Jesse had no desire to be in church on a Sunday night, but his buddy Adam had invited him, and he felt a sense of obligation. "A healing service," Jesse muttered, "during the Daytona 500?"

As the service began, the pastor asked everyone who believed in God's healing power to come forward and lay hands Darcy, a girl who had been diagnosed with leukemia. Adam went forward; Jesse remained in his seat.

The first to pray was an older woman who began in a loud voice, "Lord, we plead for the healing of this child. Make her well, Lord. Heal her of this disease. Please, God— if it is your will."

"If it is your will?" Jesse thought. "Why wouldn't it be? What kind of God would want little girls to have cancer?"

"Please, God, remove this affliction from her," the lady begged, "if you are willing."

"That's not a God I want to deal with," Jesse thought. He got up quietly and slipped out the back door.

M ost of us practice hit-and-run prayer for healing. Our technique goes something like this. First, we hear that Joe is sick, and we pray a simple prayer such as, "Dear God, you know Joe is sick. Father, you know his problem, so we ask that if it's your will for him to be healed, that you do so in the name of Jesus. Amen." And we may even anoint Joe with oil. Now if Joe doesn't get well, we have a tried-and-true dictum that explains the lack of healing. We say, "It wasn't God's will for Joe to be healed." We conclude that God must want Joe to be sick, and we go on about our business.

It is interesting that we don't apply that logic to anything else in life. If we turn a light switch into the on position and light doesn't appear, we don't conclude that the principles that govern electricity have somehow stopped working. We don't accept that we must live our lives in the dark. No, we examine the bulb or check the circuit breaker to see what the problem might be. Why don't we do that when we pray for healing?

There are far more effective ways to pray than the one described above. One reason some people are not healed is that we simply do not know how to pray effectively for them. I have stated several times that the person who most influenced my understanding of healing over two decades ago was John Wimber—a pastor and church leader in Southern California. John observed a very simple, five-step outline used effectively in praying for healing. It has been helpful to many who have desired to learn how to pray for the sick. Let's examine it.

John Wimber's Five Steps to Healing Prayer

When Jesus' disciples were unable to heal a demon-possessed boy, Jesus showed exasperation at their lack of competence (Luke 9:40–41). A parallel passage shows that after Jesus completed the healing, the disciples asked him privately how he had done it (Mark 9:28–29). When Jesus commissioned the seventy-two, he told them to do all that he had taught them to do (Luke 10:1–16). Obviously, there were techniques that the disciples could learn and use in their own ministry. I don't suggest that the following prayer techniques are the only ones that will be effective in praying for healing. Yet they are certainly more effective than the hit-and-run technique. Wimber's outline has been a tremendous help to me in praying for healing. Let it be the starting point in your ministry of healing.

1. Interview the Ailing Person

The best way to pray for the sick is with a group. It is usually a simple matter, and very nonthreatening, to simply ask the ailing person, "Where does it hurt?" Too often our prayers for healing are vague, asking God to "bless so-and-so" or stating that "God knows the need." Our prayers are more effective when we zero in on a request, asking God specifically to touch the afflicted area. Specific prayer is more effective than generalized prayer.

2. DIAGNOSE THE NEED

We're borrowing a medical term, but it is not applied to a medical condition. We don't approach the patient as if we were doctors. Yet we can try to discern any underlying factors that have caused the person to become sick. Remember that inner healing precedes physical healing. Is the person dealing with inner stresses? Are their relationships with God and others in harmony? Without giving the person the third degree, you can ask things like, "What's going on in your life right now?" Ask questions that will uncover any important issue beyond the physical symptoms that are presented.

> We often cover our lack of faith with the words "if it is your will."

If you don't ask the right questions, you can spend a lot of time going down the wrong path. Allow me to illustrate with the story of a humorous event that happened to me. I was on my way to a board meeting at Oklahoma Wesleyan University. I had just arrived at the airport in Tulsa, Oklahoma, and was expecting to be met at the airport by a student, who would drive me to the campus.

I waited nearly an hour. Finally, I called the school to see if there was a problem. I was just about to rent a car and drive to the school when a young man approached me sheepishly and asked if I was Dr. Garlow. I said I was, and he apologized profusely for being late. "You'll never believe what happened," he said.

Judging by the look on the poor fellow's face, I thought he'd had a flat tire or maybe been involved in an accident.

"It's worse than that," he assured me. My blank look prompted him to go on.

He said, "I saw you get off the plane. But I didn't know what you looked like, so I didn't know that was you. I walked up to a man that I thought might be you, and I said, 'Are you Dr. Garlow?' and he said, 'Yes,' so I took him to my car. He got in the car with me, and we drove for quite a long time. He started asking me about my classes and my major and when I would graduate."

I nodded a bit in shock.

"Then the man told me he was on his way to a meeting of the National Association of Intercollegiate Athletics. I told him that that group wasn't meeting at Oklahoma Wesleyan Univesity in Bartlesville, Oklahoma. Then he asked, 'Aren't you taking me to the Mariott in Tulsa?'"

The two were about halfway to campus when the student realized he'd picked up the wrong person. So he spun the car around and headed back to the airport.

I laughed, and asked him, "What did you guys talk about on the way back to the airport?"

He said, "Nothing. Nobody said a word."

The application to healing is obvious. You've got to ask the right questions. Do your homework. Find out what's really happening so that you can be specific when you pray. Remember that this is not an interrogation. We're motivated by love, not merely a desire to know the details of a person's life. During this interview, be asking, "Holy Spirit, show us how to pray."

3. Select the Type of Prayer to Be Used

John Wimber has stated that there are various types of prayers, and the prayer you select will depend upon what you have learned from the person for whom you are praying.

Petition. A petition is a request for a specific thing. This may be the simplest prayer—one that asks God to make the person well. This may be a short-term prayer.

Intercession. Intercession is made when God has appointed you to stand in the gap on behalf of another person. An intercessor usually takes on a longer-term responsibility to pray on behalf of an ailing person, seeing the prayer project all the way through.

Command. A command prayer is used when the Holy Spirit directs you. This type of prayer commands the power that is ours in Jesus' name. Here is an example: "I command that need to be met in the name of Jesus." This type of prayer is never used unless you have a clear sense that God is telling you to do so. When you consistently ask God for his direction in prayer, he will occasionally lead you to use this type of prayer. This prayer must spring from our close connection to the Father. If you pray this way on your own initiative, it will seem foolish. But if the Spirit of God has instructed you to make a command, it will be effective. As mentioned in chapter 19, we don't command God. We make requests of God. But we command the demonic world—by God's authority.

Rebuke. A rebuke is similar to a command in that it must be directed by the Holy Spirit. We don't take this responsibility upon ourselves. It differs in that it is directed toward the illness or the Enemy. Rebuke prayers are used in cases of demon affliction or direct involvement by the Enemy.

Pronouncement. Jesus made pronouncements on occasion, as did his disciples. A pronouncement prayer simply pronounces that a sick person is well. It is a statement of great faith before God. Like a command or rebuke, it should be used only when directed by the Holy Spirit. This may be the most rare type of prayer for healing.

Choose your prayer for healing as indicated by the situation and by watching what the Father is doing. Let God direct your healing prayer and it will be more effective.

4. EVALUATE RESULTS

When you have prayed for healing, evaluate the result. You may do that even during a time of prayer. Ask, "How are we doing? What kind of changes are you feeling?" After I pray, I always ask people who are experiencing pain to tell me the truth about their pain. I ask, "Is it the same, better, or worse?" I don't want people to say they feel better just to make me feel good. I want them to experience God's healing power. But if they haven't, I want to know.

If there are no results, ask, "God, how do you want us to pray?" Then continue to pray as long as the diseased person or the others around sense that God is moving. You may observe changes in the ill person, or you may have a sense in your spirit that something is happening. You may even feel it in your own body, a physical sensation that tells you God is present. When you see these manifestations of God's work, keep praying. Take a break if you need to. Be guided by this rule: As long as God's working, you keep working. If you sense that he has stopped, then stop.

> Small groups are the best place to begin praying for healing.

What drew me into praying for healing in 1983 was John Wimber's honesty. Previously, I had seen so much fakery that I wondered if healing was real. But when I heard Wimber and his prayer team asking ailing people "How are you doing?" and not merely assuming that they had been fully healed, I realized that what they were doing was genuine. Be honest in evaluating your results in healing prayer.

5. Give Post-Prayer Direction

We talk often about people being healed, but we seldom talk about them staying well—what people need to do to *keep* their healing and maintain their health. Yet retaining the healing is just as important as getting it. Suppose you have prayed for someone who had a sexually transmitted disease and the person was healed. At that point you would tell him to walk in moral purity so he would not suffer the disease a second time. If a person is healed from a common cold and you discover that she has been sleeping for only four hours a night, you might say, "God touched you, but you want to retain what God has done. You cannot continue as you have been and expect to stay well."

Post-prayer direction must be given sensitively. We want to encourage people to live healthy lives, not chastise them for their mistakes.

STARTING AT HOME

The ideal place to begin praying for healing using this five-step outline is in a home group. Home groups (or small groups) are a wonderful source of fellowship and a place of prayer. Every Christian should be involved in one. I know of one pastor who feels so strongly about this subject that he will not pray for the healing of an individual unless he or she is involved in a home group. Your home group is the best place to begin the practice of divine healing. It is a place where you can work with a team of people whom you know and who care about each other to release God's healing power.

LET'S PRAY

Father—

I long to communicate with you more often and more effectively. Yet, like Jesus' first disciples, I know that I must be taught to pray. Teach me to be sensitive to your Spirit and to the needs of those around me. Enable me to trust you completely and to call upon you freely.

In Jesus' name I ask this,
Amen.

For small group discussion questions on this chapter and additional resources on healing, visit www.wesleyan.org/gsh.

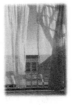

TWENTY-FOUR

WHAT SHOULD I SAY WHEN I PRAY?

When I pray God's Word,
he will watch over it to perform it.

Since she became a Christian five years ago, Rhoda Jennings had been nervous to pray aloud in groups. Everyone else's prayers seemed so eloquent and profound. "My prayers sound like a seventh grader's," Rhoda thought.

Rhoda faithfully attended prayer meeting every Wednesday. Often, members of the congregation would gather around sick or hurting people and lay hands on them.

This week Gertrude Mueller asked for prayer for herself and her eighty-seven-year-old husband.

"Rhoda," the pastor said, "would you mind praying for Herb and Gertrude?"

Rhoda's palms began to sweat and her heart raced. She had no idea what to say. "Um, sure," she stammered, then stalled for time. She fidgeted with her Bible, desperately searching for something to say. Nothing came to mind.

"Lord, please give me something to say," she prayed silently.

Rhoda looked down at her Bible, open to the Twenty-Third Psalm. She closed he eyes and began to pray. "The Lord is my shepherd, I shall not want."

M any people fumble for the right words to say in prayer, and others simply do not pray because they have no idea what to say. Perhaps even worse is the fact that some people sort of spew words, believing that the more they say, the more effective their prayers will be. So what should we say when we pray for healing? When we pray, what words should be used?

The simplest place to begin in praying for healing is to use the words that God has already given us—Scripture. Praying Scripture is an especially effective way to pray for healing, precisely because the words are not ours; they are God's. And God will watch over his Word to perform it.

KNOWING GOD'S WORD

Let's review two well-known Scripture passages and see the connection between them. Isaiah 53:4–5 says, "Surely he took up our infirmities and carried our sorrows, yet we considered him stricken by God, smitten by him, and afflicted. But he was pierced for our transgressions, he was crushed for our iniquities; the punishment that brought us peace was upon him, and by his wounds we are healed."

And Matthew 8:16–17 says, "When evening came, many who were demon-possessed were brought to him, and he drove out the spirits with a word and healed all the sick. This was to fulfill what was spoken through the prophet Isaiah: 'He took up our infirmities and carried our diseases.'"

Notice the phrase "this was to fulfill what was spoken through the prophet Isaiah." Matthew tells us that what Isaiah predicted was carried out by the ministry of Jesus. Isaiah said it, but Jesus did it. So what was so special about Isaiah? Nothing, really. He was just a man. But he was speaking the word of God. God said to Isaiah, "I want you to tell the people this." And Isaiah told them. Then, centuries later, God made sure that that word was fulfilled. That's a principle in Scripture: God watches over his Word to perform it. When God says something, he makes it happen.

> God's Word is powerful. It always accomplishes the purpose for which it was intended.

When people who know the Word of God are filled with it, and when their spirits are saturated with Scripture and they understand it, they are much more likely to pray effectively for healing.

SPEAKING GOD'S WORD

There is power in speaking. But there is greater power in speaking the Word. As mentioned earlier, Jesus once had a conversation with a centurion. The centurion wanted healing for his servant, but he insisted that Jesus didn't need to come see him. "Just say the word," the centurion told Jesus, "and my servant will be healed" (Matt. 8:8). In Mark 11:23 Jesus said, "If anyone says to this mountain. . . ."

When we speak God's Word in faith, God honors it. God watches over his Word to perform it. Jeremiah 1:12 says exactly that; he watches over his Word, and he's going to see that it happens.

When we pray for healing, we speak God's word for healing to those around us. The appendix to this book contains prayers that are drawn from Scripture. You can use these prayers to speak God's Word for healing to yourself and to those around you. Use them to begin your ministry of healing, claiming the power of the Covenant by speaking the Word of God.

> When we pray God's Word, we claim God's authority.

A caution is needed here. The principle of speaking the Word can be abused. Some people have come to believe that we can simply tell God what to do and he must do it. This abuse is popularly called the *Name It, Claim It* teaching. But we are not interested in manipulating God into giving us what we want—as if that were possible. We are talking about receiving the healing power that God has promised in his Word.

The Father is passionately in love with you, and he wants you to be well. Nothing gives him greater satisfaction than to hear his children repeat the words he has given to them. Memorize Scripture. Meditate upon it. Allow it to saturate your spirit. Then, when you need it most, recall it and speak it. Then trust God to perform his Word, as he has promised to do.

MY HEALING

I have referred several times to a respiratory ailment that I suffered some time ago. In 1992 I had developed a cough that was quite severe. On April 2 at 3:30 in the afternoon, a coughing spell came on me that was so severe that I thought I might die. I tried to get into another room of the house where Carol was, but I didn't make it.

I collapsed on the floor. The doctor later told me that I'd had a laryngeal spasm, which cut off my airway so that I couldn't breathe. After I passed out, my muscles relaxed so that I could breathe again. I was terrified about what had happened.

The same thing happened again the next morning, and from then on these spasms came upon me as often as five or six times a day. I had no more than three or four seconds notice before my airway was completely closed. Often I would begin to cry out for help and was unable to produce a sound. Finally I was confined to bed for two weeks. I was living in terror of the next spasm, never completely sure if I would wake from it.

During that time I began listening to a recording of healing songs intermixed with Bible passages on healing. I would put the tape player beside my bed at night, and I played that recording over and over throughout those long nights. God's word to King Hezekiah found in 2 Kings 20:5, was especially meaningful to me. It says, "I have heard your prayer and seen your tears; I will heal you." Each time the tape played, I waited eagerly to hear those words. They were a source of incredible comfort and strength to me. Why? Because they are God's words. And during the night hours, via cassette tape, the Word of God was spoken to me.

My healing did not come quickly. I slowly improved over the next thirteen years, and I have been free from those attacks for some time now. My healing was not instantaneous, but it did come, praise God! And a critical part of that healing was discovering the power of God's Word, spoken to me. For God's Word is powerful and effective. And he will watch over it to make it so.

LET'S PRAY

Father—
Your Word is powerful and effective, sharper than any
two-edged sword, able to penetrate the human heart, piercing

the mind and revealing hidden thoughts. And your Word is powerful and effective; I know that it will not return to you empty handed. It will accomplish the purpose for which it was sent. I ask that you will place your words into my mouth so that I may speak with authority, asking for health and healing in the name of Jesus.

Amen.

For small group discussion questions on this chapter and additional resources on healing, visit www.wesleyan.org/gsh.

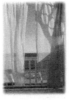

CAN IT REALLY BE TRUE THAT GOD STILL HEALS?

*We must accept by faith that which
we do not understand.*

Jan shifted uncomfortably in her seat, arms folded tightly in front of her. The four couples in her small group had just begun a six-week study on the subject of healing. Jan would have skipped the meeting—except that it was her turn to host.

"Who has a prayer request?" Jerry asked. A recital of ailments followed. Someone's aunt had suffered a stroke, a brother-in-law was facing bypass surgery, and two kids had the croup.

"OK," Jerry concluded, "Everybody grab a hand and let's ask God to heal these diseases."

Jan hesitated. Should she say what she was thinking? She thought of her mother, lying ill in the hospital. Jan's mom had been fighting cancer for two years. With each round of treatment, she had less faith that medicine would make her mother well. Was there any hope?

"Jerry," she said. "I have one more—it's my mom. I'd like us to pray for her. I want to believe God can heal her . . . I just don't know if I can."

C an it really be true that God still heals? Do we dare to believe in the things that we cannot verify scientifically? That's the bottom-line question that most people have about healing. At the end of the day, we're far less concerned with how and when God heals than we are with the basic notion that he heals at all. How can we know for sure that all of this is true? How can we be sure that God still heals?

The answer to that question has something to do with the way we understand the world and something to do with the culture in which we live. But ultimately, it is a matter of faith.

A THREE-TIERED WORLD

In the modern world we have been trained to interact with the world empirically. That simply means that we have been taught to accept as true only what we can perceive with our five senses. If we can see, hear, touch, smell, or taste it, we have no trouble believing it.

Yet we are spiritual beings, and most of us know—even if we're not taught it in school—that some things exist that we cannot experience with our five senses. Most people believe that God exists. Surveys consistently reveal that people do believe in heaven as a place where people live after they die. We know that there is a spiritual world, even though we can't see it. So most of us accept this idea that there are two worlds, a physical world and a spiritual world.

What we have more trouble with is what a professor at Fuller Theological Seminary has called the *excluded middle*. That term refers to the area of overlap between the physical and spiritual worlds. Many people who have no trouble believing in God begin to balk at the idea that God is at work in our world right now. People

> God is not distant and unconcerned. He involves himself directly in our lives.

who accept the existence of angels often find it hard to believe that an angel could appear on earth before them. Oddly, it seems to be only in the Western world that this intermixing of the physical and spiritual realms seems hard to believe.

To believe that God still heals means accepting the excluded middle, the overlap between the physical and spiritual worlds. It means believing not only that God exists but also that he is active in the world right now.

A CULTURAL PERSPECTIVE

If I were to teach on the subject of divine healing in another culture, I might not present it in the same way because people in many other cultures have less difficulty accepting the idea of supernatural involvement in the world. For example, I was preaching on healing in one of the poorest areas of Haiti. In my message I did not use most of the rationalistic arguments that I have used in this book. Why? Because most of the people there had no trouble believing that God is actually at work in the world. I simply said, "God wants to heal you."

On that night I witnessed one of the greatest healings I have ever seen. An old man was there whose legs were crippled. He came forward after I preached on healing, and I thought, "My goodness, this man can barely stand." A moment later I heard the snapping sound of his crutches hitting the floor, and I realized that the man was standing on his own two feet. People clapped and cheered as he began to walk—and then run. I confess that my faith had been weak that night, but it was strengthened by the miracle I witnessed at that moment. When the man realized that he could stand on his own, he was filled with joy and started running and leaping. He had been healed.

There was no excluded middle in that place. The people didn't need a rationalistic explanation for what they had seen. They lived in a world in which they could embrace the material and spiritual with equal ease. To us, this may seem primitive or prescientific. To them, it was reality.

THE NEED FOR FAITH

In the end we must accept by faith that which we cannot verify or fully understand. I pray that you have realized that God is establishing his Kingdom on planet earth and that that Kingdom includes the healing of sick and diseased bodies. When the full manifestation of the Kingdom comes, there will be no disease. All sickness, sorrow, and death will be gone. That will be the main course of the Kingdom banquet. For now, we have the appetizer. We see glimpses of healing, and we long for more.

> The decision to trust God for healing is an act of faith.

Where is this Kingdom that is coming? It is within you right now. I pray that you may approach this subject with childlike faith, taking Scripture at face value, taking God at his Word. You have a loving heavenly Father who longs for you to be well. It is impossible to prove that to you by empirical means, yet it is true. As you go forth to pray for the sick, may the blessings of God surround you, and may you be enabled to release God's healing power to those in need.

LET'S PRAY

Father—

I believe in you. I believe that you are real. I believe that you are good. And I believe that you reward those who earnestly seek you. I am seeking you now, Lord, for myself and for those around me. I ask for your healing power to be released in my life. I want to be healthy. Please make me well. I ask for your healing power to be released in others. I lift their names before you, calling upon your mercy. Enable me to pray faithfully and continually so that we may be well.

In Jesus' name I ask this.

Amen.

For small group discussion questions on this chapter and additional resources on healing, visit www.wesleyan.org/gsh.

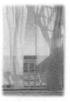

APPENDIX A

SCRIPTURE PRAYERS FOR HEALING
by Carol Jane Garlow

There is no more effective way to pray for healing than to speak God's own words in prayer. The Bible says, "So is my word that goes out from my mouth: It will not return to me empty, but will accomplish what I desire and achieve the purpose for which I sent it" (Isa. 55:11). When we pray Scripture, we claim the authority of God's Word. And it is that authority that brings results.

These prayers are based on paraphrases of various scriptures that deal with aspects of healing. Use them to begin praying for your own healing, or that of others. In time, you may begin to create your own healing prayers based on the Word of God.

FOR ABUNDANT LIFE AND WHOLENESS

Father in heaven, Your Word promises an abundant life and an everlasting covenant with You. You say to us, "Come, all you who are thirsty, come to the waters. . . . Give ear and come to me; hear me, that your soul may live. I will make an everlasting covenant with you, my faithful love promised to David. . . . Seek the LORD while he may be found; call on him while he is near. . . . For my thoughts are not your thoughts, neither are your ways my ways. . . As the heavens are higher than the earth, so are my ways higher than your ways, and my thoughts than your thoughts. . . . So is my word that goes out from my mouth: It will not return to me empty, but will accomplish what I desire and achieve the purpose for which I sent it." May these words soak into my spirit and bring forth the abundant life You so graciously extend to me. May the covenant of life I have with You, Father, accomplish the things You desire to prosper in me. I worship and give praise to You, my Lord and God. Amen.

(Paraphrased from verses in Isaiah 55)

FOR REDEMPTION AND RESTORATION

Father in heaven, I praise You for Your redemption and restoration. I do not have to fear, for You have redeemed me. You call me by my name, and You say I am Yours. When I pass through the waters of stormy, chaotic times, You will be with me. When I go through rivers, the circumstances will not overflow around me. When I walk through the fire of difficulty, I will not be burned, nor will the flame scorch me. My Redeemer says to me, " I am Your Lord, Your Holy One, the Creator of Israel, Your King." He is the One who makes a way in the sea and a path through the mighty waters. The Lord will restore health to me and heal my wounds. In the triumph of my redemption and restoration, You will pour out Your Spirit on me and my descendants. You will also send blessings upon me and my offspring. I thank You and worship You, my God. Amen.

(Paraphrased from Isaiah 43:1–2, 15–16; 44:3; Jeremiah 30:17)

FOR SEEKING GOD

Father, I come before You, blessing the name of the Lord, with praise continually in my mouth. Humbly I bow on my knees to commit my needs and desires to You. May my main desire always be to seek You, for You are near to those whose hearts are broken and whose spirits are contrite. As I quiet myself in Your presence, may Your Spirit nourish and meet the physical and spiritual needs I have. The afflictions of the righteous can have many different components, but Your Word says You will deliver me from them all. Thank You for hearing me and delivering me from all my fears. Oh Lord, how wonderful it is to taste and see how good You are. There are great blessings when I trust in You. Amen.

(Paraphrased from Psalm 34)

FOR GOD'S HEALING ANOINTING

O, give thanks to the Lord, for He is good! His mercy endures forever. Whenever I cry out to the Lord in my trouble, He saves me from my distresses. All the Lord has to do is send His Word, and He heals me. He also delivers me from the destruction of my ways. Jesus, You modeled healing for Your disciples and even sent them out to heal. Your anointing to heal still has power to bring health and wholeness for my total being—spiritually, emotionally, and physically. Thank You, Father, for the gift of healing. I sense that the presence of the kingdom of God has come near to me and to those who pray for me. I give thanks to You, Lord, for Your goodness and for the wonderful works demonstrated in my life. Amen.

(Paraphrased from Psalm 107:1, 19–21; Luke 10:9)

TO EXPRESS TRUTH AND CONFIDENCE IN GOD

Father in heaven, You know what has come upon me. The joy of my heart has ceased, and my dance has turned into mourning. Yet in my heart I have confidence that You, O Lord, remain forever. I need to turn back to You in order to be restored. Renew my days, as in the past. Thank You, O Lord, for being merciful to me. My soul trusts in You. I will make my refuge in the shadow of Your wings until these calamities have passed by. My heart is steadfast, O Lord. I love to sing and give praise, for Your mercy reaches to the heavens and Your truth reaches to the clouds. I exalt You, O Lord, above the heavens, and Your glory is above all the earth. Amen.

(Paraphrased from Lamentations 5:1, 15, 19, 21; Psalm 57:1, 7, 10–11)

FOR HEALING FROM PAIN AND DISEASE

Father in heaven, I praise You and extol You, for You have lifted me up. When I am experiencing anguish and pain, I can cry out to You, and You will heal me. Oh Lord, my body and soul feel close to death. I look to Your Word, which says, "You brought me up from the grave; you spared me from going down into the pit" (Ps. 30:3). Father, You desire to keep my spirit lifted and not in despair. My problems cause weeping that may endure for a night, but there is joy that comes in the morning. I will continue to cry out to You, O Lord, and make my supplication to You. You do hear, O Lord, and will have mercy on me and be my helper. I thank You, my God, for turning my mourning into dancing; You take my mourning clothes and wrap me with gladness. My soul sings praises to You, and it will not be silent. I know that You are the Lord my God, and I will give thanks to You forever. Amen.

(Paraphrased from Psalm 30)

FOR FORGIVENESS

Father, You are Jehovah-Rapha, the one who heals. We thank You for Your forgiving nature that cleanses us from all our sins. In forgiveness comes much healing. We place the sicknesses and disease that plague our bodies under the authority of Your Word. By the power of your Word, we declare healing over the emotional trauma and spiritual bondage that affects us. Amen.

(Paraphrased from Psalm 103:2–3 and 1 Corinthians 4:20)

TO CLAIM VICTORY THROUGH GOD'S STRENGTH

My God, Jehovah-Nissi, I declare that You are my banner, my victory. This battle of _____ that I am fighting is terrifying me. I am overcome with doubt and fear. I do not want to live day to day in discouragement and defeat. I am determined to draw strength from the promises of Your Word so that I will have courage to fight this battle. Your banner of love, victory, and guidance will go before me always. This is a time when I need to claim a mentality of victory and take a firm stand with my Jehovah-Nissi right beside me. I will not be afraid or dismayed because of this great difficulty, for the battle is not mine alone, but God's. Thank You, Father, for placing your banner of victory over my life. Amen.

(Paraphrased from Joshua 1:9 and 2 Chronicles 20:15)

FOR HEALING THROUGH THE CROSS OF CHRIST

Jesus Christ, our high priest, You are the one we can call upon to tell all that is on our hearts. You know all about our sorrows, our grief, our hurt, and our pain because You have experienced all of these things yourself. You were despised and rejected by many, and we have not always valued who You really are. In spite of all this, You, Jesus, have chosen to take upon yourself our sorrows; You will carry the burden of our hurts and our pain. What love You have for us! When we realize that the agony and suffering You endured in Your lifetime was for us, we are amazed. It is our wrongdoing, our sin and impurity that put You on a cross. It is our iniquity, our wickedness and rebellion, that wounded, crushed, and pierced You. Thank You, Lord, for Your sacrifice. Thank You for this act that brought salvation, wholeness, and an abundant and full life for all who acknowledge what You have done. This atoning work, those stripes that were laid upon You, brings us healing, divine healing. We thank and praise You, Jesus, for by faith in You, we can receive healing from our physical sicknesses. The emotional hurts in our hearts can receive healing; our minds can be renewed and healed. Again, we thank You, Jesus, for Your love, mercy, and forgiveness. Your Name is to be praised and glorified. Amen.

(Paraphrased from Isaiah 53)

FOR STRENGTH DURING PAIN AND SUFFERING

O Lord, I have waited patiently to be brought out of this horrible pit. The pain and suffering of my (sin, trauma, or sickness) makes me feel as though I am stuck in miry clay. I know that God can set my feet upon a rock; He can establish my steps. Please do not withhold Your tender mercies from me. O Lord, let Your lovingkindness and Your truth preserve me continually. Rather than dwelling in the pain and devastation that consumes me, I desire Your sustenance and strength. I want to know Jesus more and to understand the power of His resurrection. For as I stand on His victory, I can have the experience of victory over my circumstances. There is also a fellowship of suffering that I share with Jesus. He understands my sufferings. Knowing Jesus, the

Christ, gives me confidence that He who began a good work in me will complete it. So with the resilience of the Lord, I press on toward the goal, the prize of the upward call of God in Christ Jesus. Amen.

(Paraphrased from Psalm 40:1–3, 11; Philippians 1:6; 3:10, 14)

For Hope through God's Mercy and Redemption

Father in heaven, I thank You for Your mercy and redemption. My lifestyle has not always honored the truth of Your Word. I cry out to You, Lord, and You hear my plea for mercy. I cannot believe how merciful and forgiving you are. My sin and wrongdoing have left me with many difficulties I cannot fix on my own. Now I am waiting on You, Lord, and I place my hope in Your Word. May the promises and the ways of Your Word be planted in my heart and mind so I can live freely in God's abundant redemption. I know that in redemption comes the wholeness and health of both my mind and body. I desire to continually worship You, for there is great expectancy in my hope in the Lord. Amen

(Paraphrased from Psalm 130)

To Express Hope and Trust in God

O Lord, I must put my hope in You; I must put my trust in You. I have many doubts and fears. I feel desperate because I cannot accept this situation anymore. O Lord, I must put my hope and trust in Your Word. I pray that my soul will wait silently for You alone. Instead of trusting in human knowledge and opinions, I put my expectations in You. You alone are my rock and my salvation. Because You are my defense, I shall not be moved. I pray that You, the God of hope, will fill me with all joy and peace as I believe in Your Word and Your promises. May I abound in hope by the power of the Holy Spirit. Amen.

(Paraphrased Psalm 39:7, Psalm 62:5, and Romans 15:13)

For Refuge and Strength When Troubled

O Lord, my God, You are my refuge and my strength. Many times I am in trouble, and Your presence is always there helping me. You are so reliable that I do not have to fear, even though calamity is on the earth and in my home. "Though the mountains be carried into the midst of the sea; though its waters roar and be troubled; though the mountains shake with the swelling . . . There is a river" (Ps. 46:3–4 KJV). Yes, Lord, that river is a symbol of Your peaceful, comforting presence that streams over me as I walk into the holy part of Your dwelling place. When I am in the midst of that place, I cannot be moved nor shaken. You, Lord, are with me. I desire to abide in the sanctuary of Your presence, and in that safe place, I will be still. It gives me the strong assurance that You are God and will bring victory to overcome the calamity of my problems. Thank You, my God. I worship You as my refuge and strength. Amen.

(Paraphrased from Psalm 46)

FOR SAFETY AND SECURITY

O Lord Most High, when I do not feel safe and secure, I need to dwell in the secret place You provide. During an attack of _____, I can hide under the shadow of El Shaddai, the Almighty. In these times I will establish You as my refuge and my fortress. I know, my God, that I can trust You. There are those who want to catch me in a trap. Satan's devices are terrorizing me, trying to destroy me. But again, Lord Most High, I know who my refuge is. I know where I can dwell so no evil can come after me. Because the Lord understands, I have set my affection toward You; You will deliver me. Because I acknowledge You and call upon You, You, Lord will answer me and be with me in my trouble. The Lord Almighty promises to deliver me and satisfy me with long life. Unto You Lord, I give all honor and glory. Amen.

(Paraphrased from Psalm 91)

FOR HELP AND PROTECTION

O God, I am lifting my eyes up to the hills, where I know the source of my help exists. In that dwelling place, You, the creator of heaven and earth, are my guardian and caretaker. Your stand is firm enough to keep me, to preserve me. You do not sleep, so I know You will always be there protecting me. Your shade protects me twenty-four hours of the day. Because I call You my Lord, you will physically and spiritually preserve and keep me from all evil. You, Lord, will guard and keep me when I go out, and You will guard and keep me when I come in, even now and throughout eternity. Praise and thanksgiving be unto You. Amen.

(Paraphrased from Psalm 121)

FOR RELIEF FROM ANXIETY

Father in heaven, I rejoice in You. Again I rejoice, for I can come to you in prayer, presenting all my requests to You. I do not have to be anxious, because I can express both my deeply felt needs and my thanksgiving to You. I pray for Your peace, which surpasses all understanding, to guard my heart and mind in the name of Jesus. I desire to fix my thoughts on You and to meditate on those things that are true, noble, just, pure, lovely, and of good report. I know I can do all things through Jesus, who has the power to give me strength and sustain me through difficult times. That which I need will be supplied according to the riches of Your creation, and You will provide abundantly according to the Your riches in glory, through Jesus Christ. Now to my God and Father, be glory forever and ever. Amen.

(Paraphrased from Philippians 4:4, 6–8, 13, 19–20)

TO EXPRESS TRUST IN GOD'S FAITHFULNESS

O Lord, my trust is in You. You encourage me to do good. There is security in dwelling in You and feeding on Your faithfulness. In You, O Lord, I can delight myself, and You will give me the desires of my heart. I can calm the anxiety I have because of this difficult situation by resting in You and waiting patiently for Your hand to do its work. Your Word promises that the salvation of the righteous is from the Lord; You are my strength in a time of trouble. I thank You, Lord, that You help me, deliver me, and save me because I trust in You. Amen.

(Paraphrased from Psalm 37)

To Request God's Provision

Father in heaven, You are worshiped, for I consider that the Lord is great and greatly to be praised. In my worship I will meditate on the glorious splendor of Your majesty and on Your wondrous works. For You, Lord, are gracious and full of compassion, slow to anger, and great in mercy. At times my life is so difficult that I feel as though I cannot make it. My steps falter, and I begin to fall. But You, Lord, come along and hold me up. When my work, my sickness, my poverty—financial or spiritual—pulls me down, You are there to raise me up. My eyes look expectantly to You because You are my ultimate source, the one who gives me all that I need in due season. You open Your hand and satisfy the desire of every living thing. Because the Lord is righteous in all His ways and gracious in all His works, I can call on Him and He will be near me. I praise and thank the Lord, for when He hears my cry, He will come and save me. I have a promise from the Word of God that says He will preserve those who love Him (Ps. 145:20). Therefore, my mouth wants to continually praise the Lord. Amen.

(Paraphrased from Psalm 145)

To Express Hope through Persistent Prayer

Father in heaven, I am in anguish. My strength and my hope have perished. In my affliction and roaming, my soul still remembers You and is bowed down within me. But I recall to my mind that I have hope. Through the Lord's mercies, I am not consumed, for His compassion does not fail. It is new every morning. I can say, "Great is your faithfulness . . . The LORD is my portion; therefore, I will wait for him" (Lam. 3:23–24). Lord, You are good to those who wait for You, to those who seek after You. Good things come my way as I wait expectantly and hope for the salvation of the Lord. Blessed be Your name! Amen.

(Paraphrased from Lamentations 3:18–26)

To Express the Power and Authority of God's Word

Jesus, thank You for coming into this world as a light shining in the darkness of evil. Satan is having a heyday with my life. I ask in

Your name to shine light into Satan's evil deeds and expose the deceit and lies. In Jesus' name I say, "Satan, get behind me! I shall only worship the Lord my God, and Him only shall I serve. I speak to you in the authority of Jesus' name that you have no hold over me, my situation, or my family. You have no authority to operate in my life, and you have no power to hurt me." Jesus, I acknowledge that You are the One whom God sent to the world because You loved us so much. I stand on the truth of God's Word and His ways. I desire the light of Jesus to shine on my life so I will be able to walk victoriously. I speak the power of God's Word to protect my life and my family. I thank You, Jesus, for the power and authority that is stronger than Satan's devices. I worship only You, who reign mightily over all areas of my life. Amen.

(Paraphrased from John 3:19, 20; Luke 4:8; 10:19; and Ephesians 5:8, 9)

TO PREPARE FOR SPIRITUAL WARFARE

Father in heaven, You give us strength in You and in the power of Your might as we go on the offensive against Satanic forces. You also give us armor that enables us to stand against the wiles of the devil. We know that the turmoil and fighting that we face is not against other people but comes from the wickedness of Satan and his demonic forces and from his power that rules in the heavenly places. In order to withstand the evil that would overwhelm us, we must put on the armor of God and simply take a stand. When we are standing, we have the truth of God's Word fastened around our waist and a breastplate of righteousness protecting the upper body. Our feet are prepared and ready, covered with the gospel of peace. We have the shield of faith as an important protection from the fiery darts of Satan's devices. The helmet of salvation on our heads encompasses our total being—spirit, body, and soul. The sword of the Spirit, which is the Word of God, give us the strength of our battle stance. And now, Satan, we speak to you. You are defeated in the name of Jesus. You have no authority over us and the problems that we face. We claim victory for this battle against _____. Thank You,

Father, for the heavenly hosts who fight with us in this battle. You are to be worshiped, praised, and honored as the one and only true God. Amen.

(Paraphrased from Ephesians 6:10–18)

FOR STRENGTH TO FIGHT BATTLES

O Lord, I will praise You with my whole heart for Your loving kindness and Your truth. When I cried out, You answered me and made me bold, with strength in my soul. Though I walk in the midst of trouble, You will be there to revive me. You will stretch out Your hand against the wrath of my enemies, and Your right hand will save me. The Lord will accomplish the healing work that concerns me. Thank You for fulfilling all the promises you have made to me and all the plans You have for my life. Your mercy, O Lord, endures forever. Amen.

(Paraphrased from Psalm 138:1–3, 7–8)

TO CLAIM VICTORY THROUGH WORSHIP

Blessed be the Lord my Rock, who trains my hands for war and my fingers for battle. Because of Your lovingkindness and compassion, I will keep my eyes on You. I will not give up, for You are my fortress, my high tower, and my deliverer. I feel Your shield about me. You are the One in whom I take refuge. I will love You, O Lord, my strength. You, Lord, are my rock. You are my God, my strength in whom I will trust. You are my shield and the horn of my salvation; You are my stronghold against Satan's plans to harm me. I will call upon the Lord, who is worthy to be praised.

(Paraphrased from Psalm 144:1, 2; Psalm 18:1–3)

FOR RELEASE FROM BURDENS AND AFFLICTIONS

Father, I come to You with the heavy burden of this affliction. I humbly submit a pure and contrite spirit to You so that in fasting and prayer, You will loose the bonds of wickedness, affliction, and disease, and undo these heavy burdens. I want Your presence and strength with me during this time. You take pleasure in the sacrifice and denial of my body and spirit as I fast, for Your power, Father, is released through this process to break the bondages. Your Word then promises that "light will break forth like the dawn and your healing will quickly appear" (Isa. 58:8). I ask for Your righteousness to go before me and for the glory of the Lord to be my rear guard. I need strength for my bones and refreshing water to rush through my spirit. I thank You, Lord, for satisfying my soul in the dry times and for guiding me continually through this experience. You are truly an awesome God. Amen.

(Paraphrased from Isaiah 58)

FOR BREAKING GENERATIONAL SINS AND CURSES

Father in heaven, I desire to break the power of generational sin and iniquity that keeps me from victory over the difficult situations in my life. The fathers and mothers in my generational line have sinned and are no more, but I bear their iniquities. First, I want to come before You, Lord, with clean hands and a pure heart. I confess those sins that have a hold on me and ask for Your forgiveness. Thank You for being faithful and just to forgive me and cleanse me from all unrighteousness. I know the generational sins that are at work in my family, and I renounce their work in my life. I forgive my ancestors for bringing sin and iniquity into the family line. Through the act of forgiving my family, the curses of these sins are beginning to break in the power of Jesus' name. They no longer have authority to operate in my life. I plead that the blood of Jesus, shed on the cross for each of my sins and the sins of the family, be appropriated into our bloodline where each sin has been committed. I renounce those sins and curses in my family line. Satan, in the name of Jesus, you have no hold or legal right to continue tormenting me, my family, my children, and the generations to come. Thank You, Father, for ruling and reigning over me. As for me and my family, we now shall receive blessings from the Lord and not curses, and we shall receive righteousness for future generations from the God of our salvation. Amen.

(Paraphrased from Lamentations 5:7; Psalm 24:4–5; 1 John 1:9; Galatians 3:13; Matthew 26:28)

FOR BLESSING UPON MY LIFE

Father in heaven, I come before You, acknowledging that You are the Lord my God. Your Word says that if I obey Your voice and observe Your commandments, blessings shall come upon me. I shall be blessed wherever I am and wherever I go. When enemies rise against me, the Lord will defeat them—not just in one way, but in seven ways. So, Father, I ask for blessings upon the work of my hands so I will be productive and have plenty. Bless the relationships in my family so that we may give love, honor, and respect in the right proportions to each other. I desire that each person in my family realize their full potential before God. I desire to worship and love You, proclaiming You Lord over my life, my family, and my church. Your Word says that You shall establish me and my family as a holy people to yourself if we walk in Your ways. Therefore, You will bless us in the physical and spiritual place You are giving to us. You will also bless us with health and good treasure as we give worship and praise to You. I declare unto You: "Worthy is the Lamb who was slain, to receive power and wealth and wisdom and strength and honor and glory and praise" (Rev. 5:12). Amen.

(Paraphrased from Deuteronomy 28:1–14 and Revelation 5:12)

TO WORSHIP GOD

Lord Jehovah, Creator of Heaven and Earth, Redeemer, Lord of Hosts, You are the First and the Last. You are the Lord, and there is no other; there is no God besides You. The Lord reigns over the heavens and the earth. He is clothed with majesty, and the heavens declare the glory of God. The firmament shows His handiwork. The earth is the Lord's and all its fullness. The Lord is my light and my salvation. He is my rock, my fortress, and my deliverer. He is my strength, my shield, and my stronghold. We will extol You, our God, and bless Your name forever. Great are You, Lord Jehovah. Amen.

(Paraphrased from various phrases in the Psalms)

FOR ANOINTING UPON THOSE
WHO MINISTER HEALING

Father in heaven, You have called and gifted me to minister salvation and emotional and physical healing to the people You place in
my path. I humbly desire that "the Spirit of the Sovereign LORD [be]
on me, because the LORD has anointed me to preach good news to the
poor; He has sent me to bind up the brokenhearted, to proclaim freedom for the captives, and release from darkness for the prisoners; to
proclaim the year of the LORD's favor and the day of vengeance of
our God, to comfort all who mourn, and provide for those who grieve
in Zion—to bestow on them a crown of beauty instead of ashes, the
oil of gladness instead of mourning, and a garment of praise instead
of a spirit of despair. They will be called oaks of righteousness, a
planting of the LORD for the display of his splendor." I pray for
strength and wisdom to be Your servant. Thank You, Father, for the
opportunity to take part in Your kingdom's work. Blessed be Your
name. Amen.

(Quoting Isaiah 61:1–3)

APPENDIX B

BLOCKAGES TO DIVINE HEALING

"If God still heals, then why isn't everyone healed?" That may be the most commonly asked question about divine healing. Here are eighteen common problems—I call them *blockages*—that can prevent people from receiving divine healing. Because we live in a fallen world, there are many cases in which we simply do not know why a person is not healed. Therefore, we should be extremely hesitant to identify blockages to healing in the lives of others. Yet understanding and removing blockages can be a key to experiencing divine healing in our own lives.

The chapter or chapters in which each blockage (or the positive factors related to it) is discussed are noted in parentheses.

1. Lack of prayer for healing.	(Chapters 15 and 17)
2. Lack of persistence in prayer.	(Chapter 21)
3. Lack of knowledge about how to pray for healing.	(Chapters 23 and 24)
4. Lack of faith on the part of the sick person.	(Chapter 14)
5. Lack of faith on the part of those praying for the sick.	(Chapter 14)

6. Sin in the life of the sick person. (Chapter 12)

7. Sin in the life of those praying
   for the sick. (Chapter 12)

8. Lack of understanding about
   spiritual authority. (Chapter 16)

9. Lack of exercising spiritual authority. (Chapter 16)

10. Lack of knowing the Word. (Chapter 24)

11. Lack of speaking the Word. (Chapter 24)

12. Lack of fasting. (Chapter 17)

13. Lack of faithful participation in
    worship, personal devotions, or
    the Lord's Supper. (Chapters 13 and 22)

14. Living an unhealthy lifestyle. (Chapter 18)

15. Not seeing what the Father is doing. (Chapter 8)

16. Inability to identify the need for
    inner healing. (Chapter 11)

17. Inability to identify familial spirits. (Chapter 20)

18. Inability to identify demonic activity. (Chapter 19)

I have identified eighteen blockages; there may be more. Yet this list is not a formula and should not be used as one. It is a guideline only.

I began this book by stating that I do not fully understand healing. I end with the same humble admission. Yet there are certain things of which I am convinced, a few nonnegotiable imperatives that apply to prayer for healing. First, love people, and never condemn. Second, pray for them. Healing occurs less often when people pray little for healing. Third, do not judge. The list above should never be used for announcing blockages. It is for pondering. Fourth, do not become discouraged when healing doesn't occur. Someone has said, "Let us not become weary in well doing." Certainly, that applies to prayer for healing. Fifth, do not allow guilt to come upon you when the healing for which you have prayed does not occur. Finally, do not allow condemnation to come upon you for any failure to pray for others in the past. You have the present. Steward it wisely.

And now may the God who loves you anoint you to lovingly and discerningly pray for the sick. Amen.

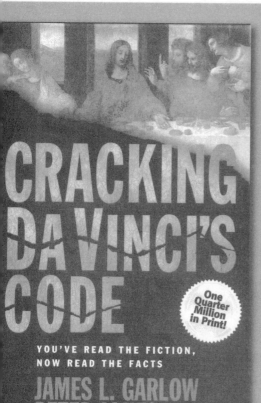

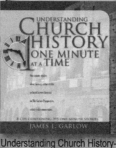
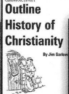